UNMASK
Your
Beauty

A transformational journey to exposing the hidden truth about you

ADEDOYIN OMOTARA

UNMASK *Your Beauty*

Published By: AWM Books
PO Box 18043 Shawnessy PO
Calgary AB, Canada T2Y 0K3
www.awmpublishing.ca

Printed in the United States

UNMASK *Your Beauty*

A transformational journey to exposing the hidden truth about you

By Adedoyin Omotara

Endorsements

Unmask Your Beauty is a must-read for any woman looking for strength and encouragement to unmask herself and break free from fear, self-doubt, and 'what will people say' syndrome. Doyin has done an excellent job guiding us gently, step by step, to the place where we can stand on our own two feet, comfortable in our skin, and fulfill our dreams and vision. Well done, Doyin!

Dee Adekugbe, President, All Woman Ministry

The *Unmask Your Beauty* book is ideal for women. The book provides you with a framework to plan out what you want your future to look like. Personally, this book helped me realize why I had succeeded in some things in the past, and why I was not able to excel on certain projects I had embarked on in the past. I would strongly recommend this book to everyone, both men and women.

Femi Omotara, Family Physician

Unmask Your Beauty is a book for the woman who wants to live a beautiful life. Doyin shares her authentic journey of unmasking her own beauty with lots of lessons you can apply to your own life. Doyin has been able to clearly put together keys that every woman needs to unearth the beauty within her, that can help her be the person she was born to be, and influence and transform the nation she has been called to. So, what you are reading in this book is not fluff or theory but practical strategies. If you want to dig deeper into who you really are and impact your nation, get yourself a copy of *Unmask Your Beauty* and start using the keys Doyin has generously shared.

Detola Amure, Productivity & Transformational Coach

I am so excited to write this review as this is not an average book, but this is a book that is an EMPOWERMENT TOOL to encourage all women, and honestly, I believe that many men will also be encouraged after reading this book. I could not put it down until I had finished! ***Unmasking Your Beauty*** is what Doyin's signature is. This book is as authentic as the writer, and it will leave you full of the possibilities of confidence, potential, and embracing your inner beauty.

Nicole Ragguette, Owner, Royal Ambassador Cleaning

Unmask Your Beauty is a must-read! It is a God-inspired manual for every woman who wants to step into her calling and live a life of purpose. It is beautifully written, captivating, and inspiring. Adedoyin captures the essence of every *"Adoniaa"* woman as she takes us on a journey of self-discovery, personal growth, and manifestation. I wholeheartedly believe that through this book, many women will be empowered to take off the masks that have hidden their true identities for so long and be liberated to birth their dreams and visions.

Mosope Idowu, Founder, Bethel Fit Mum

Adedoyin went through a deep and fulfilling process of self-discovery, birthing the vision for her personal brand and her business, Adoniaa, in the process. She has very generously documented the process with very detailed exercises at the end of each chapter to help us navigate our way to our individual self-discovery. A common theme running through the book is the evidence of her deep relationship with God and how beneficial her knowing Him has been to her. I am confident this book is just a scratch on the surface of a series of books coming from this powerhouse of a woman. I look forward to them all.

Damilola Ajibade
Founder, Crownbury and International Tax Consultant

Contents

CHAPTERS

Dedication

Dedicated to all Adoniaa women who dare to embrace the truth of who they are and use their God-given talents and abilities, realizing that God created us all for a unique purpose.

ii

Acknowledgment

To my darling Lord and Savior, words are not enough to express how much I love and adore you. Thank you for choosing me to do your work. In you and with you, I am deeply fulfilled. I love you, Abba, Father.

Olufemi, my Babyluv, lover, and best friend, thank you for going on this visionary ride with me. Thank you for believing in my dreams and making them yours. Thank you for sound leadership. I love all of you!

Adeoluwa and Olurotimi, my two nations, thank you for supporting me in writing this book. Thank you for always making me a proud mum. I love you both dearly.

To my parents, thank you for raising and nurturing me in the way of the Lord. Thank you for praying for me always. I feel your prayers every single day. I love you.

To my amazing coaches, Detola Amure and Debola Deji-Kurunmi, thank you for being the perfect mid-wives to birth the visions God has given me. Thank you for praying for and with me. Thank you for the gift that you are to the world. I love you both.

To my sisters and brother, thank you for cheering me on and praying for me always. What will I do without you all in my life?

To Dee Adekugbe and the entire AWM Publishing House team, thank you for your mentorship, your advice, and, most importantly, for holding my hands through the publishing process of this book.

Thank you, Seun Ibiyemi of the Super Working Mum Academy, for helping with the editing of this book and for giving constructive feedback throughout the process.

Thank you to all my amazing friends and *Adoniaa women* around the world. Thank you for believing and supporting my dream. I love you all.

Foreword

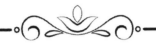

*U*nmask Your Beauty is a heartfelt masterpiece for any woman seeking to discover and rediscover her true essence, authentic identity, and God-given purpose in a refreshing way. From the moment I met Adedoyin in a coaching relationship, I was drawn to her personality, genuineness, and wisdom. Every single session with her had me so excited about her powerful vision, refreshing spirituality, and burning passion for making a difference for others. She loves herself, her work, and the world around her!

For sure, the author of this book has not merely written for authorship's sake. Adedoyin has poured out her heart in this brilliant manual because she is herself a recipient of its insights.

Within *Unmask your Beauty*, you will find yourself—both who you are right now and who you can be as you evolve into MORE. The beautiful thing is that MORE means different things to each of us as

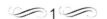

women, and this book, I hope, helps you clarify what growth would look like for you.

Written in storytelling style and delivered with excellent clarity; this book leads you on a journey of peeling off the layers of societal expectations, labels, and past pains or pretense; as you go deeper to unveil the real you - full of strength, success, and significance. No matter how long it has taken you, you are here now. You will see through *Unmask Your Beauty* that the future you seek begins from within, and the moment you wake up is your own morning!

I invite you to step into this amazing treasure hunt that will help you rediscover yourself, find your purpose, step out with your assignment and begin to create your dream life through the power of a compelling vision. Destiny awaits, and this is a fresh start for you! Congratulations.

Debola Deji-Kurunmi,
Founder, IMMERSE Coaching Company

Introduction

Growing up, I had an idea of what my life should look like based on my upbringing and what society promoted: go to school, get a job, get married, have kids, build my career, retire and eventually die!

There was no room in my head to think about any other way of doing life. It was a vision I carried with so much conviction from childhood, and nothing was going to stop me from passing through each of these stages as they were clearly defined in my mind. I practically lived my life this way until I got to the career-building stage of my beautifully planned life and realized that there was way more to life than these stages I had allowed society to define for me.

I remember vividly the feeling I had on my 26th birthday. I felt I was living the life with all I had achieved. I had an engineering degree, an amazing husband, a beautiful baby boy, a great job working as an IT consultant at a multinational company. Life was so good!

I asked myself, "how much better can life get?" I felt I had worked twenty-six long years to achieve all of this. I celebrated myself with a pink dress from Debenhams (a UK department store), went to dinner with my family, and ultimately felt a sense of fulfillment. I still remember that feeling of excitement like I was getting this life thing and living up to the standard.

Not long after, I started feeling disengaged with myself, and I just felt like this was not my best. It was as if everything inside of me was shouting, "Use me! Use me! Use me!" I felt I had so much more to offer, so much more in me that I had not expressed. There had to be more. There had to be more to life than all the things I had achieved, but I was unsure how to get to the more. And then I started to ask myself these three questions:

1) ***Who am I?*** I wanted to be clear on who I was as I found myself just doing things based on a set standard. I was hitting my goals, friends and family were proud of me, and I had even helped people land their first jobs, but something just did not feel right. It was as if there was a disengagement between my successes and who I truly was at my core.

2) ***Why am I here on earth?*** I also started to think, how am I sure this is what I should be doing? I realized that I was not completely happy with my job. It did not give me any fulfillment apart from the money I was earning. I started to

question what my purpose was and if my line of career was where I belonged.

3) *Where am I going with all these achievements?* I questioned myself about where I was going with all my accomplishments. At that time, I had an engineering degree, several IT and project management certifications, because I was particularly good at passing exams. But I was getting tired of this goal-oriented living and began asking myself what dreams I had for my future. What did all these achievements matter in the larger context of things?

These questions were so deep, and I could not figure out the answers to them; therefore, I continued with my life. Everybody seemed to think I was doing well, oblivious to the way I was feeling. The disengagement continued, and I often found myself asking the same questions repeatedly. I found these questions difficult because my parents could not answer them for me; neither could my husband or any doctor, professor, or pastor. The questions were so frightening that I just decided to blank out that part of my brain whenever they arose because I could not answer them.

Nevertheless, as I could not answer these questions, I decided the job I was doing was too simple. Maybe changing roles would make me feel more fulfilled in life, and I would eventually experience the more that I had been craving. Consequently, I changed to professional roles that I felt would challenge me—thinking that would bring me fulfillment.

I remember feeling so happy and ready to conquer the world during the first six months into my new role. Still, after a while, I began feeling that lack of motivation again and started seeking more. The old feeling had returned. This feeling continued until I realized that switching roles and getting more challenging positions in different companies was not the solution. I was not happy with the woman I was, but neither was I super clear on who I wanted to become.

After building an IT career in the oil and gas industry for several years, I realized that was not the direction I wanted to go. So, I decided to explore entrepreneurship. Maybe it would give me the more that I so yearned for. I asked myself, what could I efficiently do as an entrepreneur? The answer was not far-fetched as I had a love for the beauty industry, especially makeup artistry. It had always been my side job, and I enjoyed it so much, but I had never fully committed to it because I felt it would not be financially sustainable. And it just did not feel like it was real work. I undervalued it at that time.

Nonetheless, in the beauty industry, I admired Tara Fela-Durotoye (popularly known as TFD), a Nigerian beauty entrepreneur who pioneered the makeup profession in Nigeria by setting up international standard makeup studios and establishing the first-ever makeup school in Nigeria. Tara had also created her beauty line of products and used it to empower young makeup artists by training them to become distributors for her brand, thereby enabling them to make money on the side. I remember the first time I went to her studio in Victoria Island, Lagos, Nigeria, to register to become a distributor as a young adult in 2008. I was so wowed by how she built an institution from something that could easily be homogeneous, like makeup. I believe that was what planted the seed of owning a sustainable beauty business in me. Still, I did not know how to manifest it, so I continued on the career path that I knew until 2014 when the thought came to me again, and I decided to explore entrepreneurship.

The Genesis of the Name

In September 2014, I started toying with the idea of building a business in the beauty industry. I remembered TFD's business, and this inspired me to become a makeup artist and build it into an institution by creating my product line. I took a bold step and registered my company and started researching labs that could make my products.

I had so much fun finding a meaningful name for my brand. I remember telling my beautiful friend, Ebinehita, of my joy at combining all the names in my family to create a name for my beauty brand. She smiled and advised me to come up with a name that reflected why I started the business. That was the first time I thought about why I wanted to create a beauty business. After some deep thinking, I knew that deep

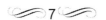

within me, I wanted women to feel more confident with themselves. The confidence theme has run through every season of my life. My friends would often ask how I exuded so much confidence in everything I did, especially in securing high paying roles. One of my friends asked how I had the confidence to apply for my last position, and I told her that once I read the job description and understood that I could perform 60 -70% of the work, I believed that the role was for me because I could learn the remaining 30 - 40% on the job.

> Our business is to make women look and feel beautiful so they can be confident to confront their fears.
>
> Adedoyin Omotara

I knew that many women would not go for jobs if they did not meet all the requirements, not me! I had something within me that most women wanted but did not know how to achieve. After going through that analysis, I concluded that beauty was confidence, beyond just makeup and skincare. When I felt really beautiful, I exuded confidence.

As much as I loved the polished look I helped women achieve by applying makeup to their faces and by teaching them how to do their makeup—something in me told me to help women polish their hearts too, not only their faces. So, for the very first time, I wrote down the reason I was starting my beauty business: *"To make women look and feel beautiful so they can be confident to confront their fears."*

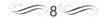

The statement sounded so profound to me because I was not sure how to achieve it. But I was persuaded that this was what I wanted to see in women, and this was my reason for wanting to start a beauty business and not any other company. I am grateful to Ebinehita for helping me kick off this meaningful dream, even when I did not understand entrepreneurship.

After coming up with why I wanted to start the business, I immediately started researching with my husband and my sister, Tomilayo, who lived with us at the time. I remember an afternoon in our conservatory in Aberdeen, Scotland, where we started to brainstorm names that reflected the above why statement. We began to Google "one word for a woman that looks and feels beautiful," and a variety of names came up, but we ended up with the name *Adoniaa* (pronounced ah-dohn-yah). *Adoniaa* is a Greek word that means a beautiful goddess or beautiful woman. My husband and sister loved the name because apart from the meaning that aligned with my why, it also sounded remarkably close to my name - *Adedoyin*, so it was easy to decide on it. The word *"Adoniaa"* carried a lot of weight for me beyond looks, and I wanted to take women on a journey of beauty beyond looks. The name led to the creation of the slogan, *"Unmask Your Beauty."*

Introduction

The Canada Move

At that time, we lived in Aberdeen, Scotland, UK, where I worked as a project planning manager but had started to process our Canadian Permanent Residency application to relocate to Canada. My plan was to create products made in Canada since we were going to live there eventually. From my research, I knew Canadians loved their country and loved to support locally made products, so I decided to support the economy by making my products in Canada.

My ultimate goal was to build the business to a point where I could leave my job and focus entirely on it. As God would have it, a year after I started my business in Aberdeen, we became permanent residents of Canada and decided to relocate. I resigned from my job and was free to focus on my business full time.

In September of 2015, we relocated to Canada. We knew only one of my old high school friends, Damilola Adamson, who came to pick us up from the airport and made dinner available the night we landed. I am still forever thankful to her for giving us a great welcome to the city of Calgary. I was so excited about the new business that I quickly started to grow my network in Calgary. I decided to try running my business full time; I planned to focus on it for two years, and if it did not work out, I would go back to my career. I came up with this Plan B because business was new to me, and I was unsure if I was making the right decision. The doubts were there.

Fast-forward. It felt so good to create a brand from scratch that I finally felt this was it. I went for a 6-month business course delivered by Momentum Calgary to fill in the knowledge gap I had, especially around entrepreneurship. I mainly wanted to learn about running a business in Canada since this was my first attempt at running a structured company. I was doing this course alongside working as a makeup artist with a few modeling agencies, and I also had my private clients. I also went on a lab tour around Canada to find a lab that could create cosmetics for every shade of woman and effective skincare for various skin conditions. I eventually found a few labs that I could work with to produce skincare and cosmetics. I gradually started testing products on myself and my clients until I could narrow down to specific skincare products, lip shades, foundation shades, powder shades, and eyeshadow colors.

The big day finally came to officially launch *Adoniaa Beauty*'s line of products on September 11, 2016, exactly a year after relocating to Canada. I was super excited, I invited the few friends I had at that time, and my friends also invited people in their networks. The hall was full of amazing women who came to support me on that day. I did not know many of them, but thanks to Ehi Ade-Mabo, Amen Adebayo, and Mosope Idowu, who filled the venue with people from their various networks.

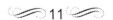

The launch event was themed *"Unmask Your Beauty,"* and because of my belief that every woman is beautiful, I did not want professional models to model my products; I wanted everyday women. I worked with some fantastic makeup artists who volunteered their time and helped pick models randomly from the guests at the launch party to showcase the *Adoniaa* makeup line.

They selected women of different races, colors, shapes, and sizes from the audience. As the women walked on the runway to showcase their makeup, I asked them what beauty meant to them. We received different answers. Some said:

"Beauty is confidence."

"Beauty is who I am."

"Beauty is showing up for yourself and other people."

"Beauty is shining your inner light."

"Beauty is ..."

The answers were powerful and insightful and gave new meaning to the word beauty.

These statements simply confirmed that beauty had a deeper meaning to women than was portrayed in the media. It felt so good to connect with women on this profound level; to see women inspired to follow their dreams and radiate the beauty that they possessed inside of them. The event ended with people trying out and buying products. I felt a great sense of achievement that night and finally thought, "Yes ... I've got this!"

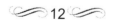

Introduction

After the product launch, I got several emails from guests about how inspired they were to go after their dreams because of what I was doing with the *Adoniaa* brand. The emails touched me. I felt I was finally bringing my vision to life.

Feeling and looking are two different things.

Adedoyin Omotara

Shortly after this, I started getting confused about integrating this more profound meaning of beauty into my makeup and beauty line and was unsure how to proceed with marketing after the launch. I no longer felt comfortable with the marketing plan I had created in business school because I had based it on my competitors' research, and I did not want to imitate them. I did not feel it was authentic enough to my vision of making women feel beautiful. It only captured a part of my dream of making women look beautiful. Feeling and looking are two different things, and I wanted to integrate them into the *Adoniaa* brand.

I started to feel an unease within me, although I knew that I was beginning to love the entrepreneurial journey, and I loved the message that was impressed upon me to share with women through beauty. This time, I was sure the solution was not to switch jobs or careers.

The unease that I felt within me caused me to start questioning myself again.

· *Who am I in all of these? What is my true identity, and how does this relate to what I am currently doing?*

· *Why am I here? What is my purpose? Is this really what I should be doing?*

· *How do I get to this future I see for women? I saw myself helping women gain more confidence but did not know how to get there.*

This time, I desperately wanted answers and decided to do something about it.

Birthing the Vision

I got in touch with a life & productivity coach named Detola Amure, who was mentoring and coaching my friend, who was in the same confusing season of life that I was in at the time. Hoping to get some answers from her, Detola made me realize that the answers to my questions were within me, and she could not give me any answers. However, she asked me questions that led me onto the path of clarity and told me that I needed to connect to the One who created me. The One who is my manufacturer, with Him alone, lies the blueprint of my life, and only He can make me understand who I am and why I have the interests that I have.

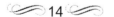

I spent the following three months after my product launch in hibernation, seeking the face of God. I was very deliberate about what I was thinking and about guarding my energy, so I stayed away from social media. My friends were worried about me because they expected me to be blasting social media with my new products and

> It is one thing to have a vision; it is another thing to know how to execute it.
>
> Adedoyin Omotara

promoting them. But I did not want to put out empty posts or copy the posts that I had seen other beauty brands posting. I wanted to be authentic and true to my vision, so I remained still to hear from God. It is one thing to have a vision; it is another thing to know how to execute it.

I also signed up for another coaching program with my friend, Curline Lyons, who had recently become a life coach. She practically said the same thing Detola had told me, to connect with the One who created me, as only He could give me the answers to those questions. I continued to work with both coaches for about three months.

During the three months of working with my coaches, fasting from social media and other distractions, I wrestled with God like Jacob in the Bible, asking Him to direct me and give me answers concerning my life and the business I was preparing to start. I was not going to leave His presence until I got answers.

One afternoon during my three months of hibernation, I was in my kitchen, cutting some spinach to make a spinach stew (Efo-riro in my Nigerian Yoruba language) when I experienced an unforgettable encounter with the Holy Spirit. (as a side note, *my spinach stew recipe is the best. You should try it!*)

Unmasking Your Beauty is to expose the true character or hidden truth about yourself.

Adedoyin Omotara

I heard in my spirit, *"Change the names of your products to the words that capture the intentions of God's heart for women. Use words that define how God created women in His image and how He wanted women to feel and to be. Use words that will help renew women's identity, that will free them of labels, and represent the truth of God's concern for women."*

Whoa! Whoa! Whoa! What a liberating day that was. It was as if somebody removed a mask from my face, and I started to see clearly. God finally helped me uncover what it truly means to *Unmask Your Beauty – "To expose the true character or hidden truth about yourself."*

I instantly felt the Spirit of God upon me, and a scripture came to mind explaining the assignment He was giving me for women regarding beauty.

Introduction

*"The Spirit of the Lord is on me because He has
anointed me to proclaim good news to the poor. He
has sent me to proclaim freedom for the prisoners
and recovery of sight for the blind, to set the
oppressed free."*
Luke 4:18 (NIV)

In my case, the prisoners, the blind, and the oppressed were women that had masked identities. Women that have forgotten who they are because of their life experiences, societal and cultural conditioning, etc. The assignment became clear to me.

I felt so liberated. I began to understand that the interest God gave me in the beauty and makeup world was really to build a platform where I could easily connect with women. To help women see their authentic, unique, and individual beauty, to see their identity clearly as God saw them, to set women free from their identity issues.

On my kitchen island that day, the Holy Spirit downloaded seventy-two qualities that genuinely exposed the hidden truth about women and the identity God had for them. I took out my journal and wrote:

*I am love, I am worthy, I am unique, I am valuable,
I am enough, I am beautiful, I am confident, I am
bold, I am limitless, I am deserving, I am capable, I
am magnificent, I am powerful, I am courageous, I
am light, I am authentic, I am strong, I am
brilliant, I am generous, I am talented, I am*

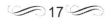

*fabulous, I am gifted, I am excellent, I am
awakened, I am joy, I am a voice, I am free, I am
fearless, I am audacious, I am an inspiration, I am
adorable, I am optimistic, I am empowered, I am
growing, I am rich, I am expressive, I am amazing,
I am mindful, I am delightful, I am
unapologetically me, I am thankful, I am ambitious,
I am grateful, I am passionate, I am positive, I am
radiant, I am righteous, I am trustworthy, I am
flourishing, I am daring, I am refreshed, I am
intelligent, I am wise, I am kind, I am whole, I am
happy, I am a creative, I am wealthy, I am blessed,
I am graceful, I am self-assured, I am connected, I
am productive, I am complete, I am a gift, I have
positive energy, I have influence, I have
abundance, I listen to my inner truth, I have peace,
I have fire in me, I unmask my beauty daily.*

I reread the words and realized that they had so much depth.
They represented how God wants us to see ourselves and, ultimately,
how He wants us to change our world by realizing who we indeed are.
So powerful.

Right there and then, I redefined beauty to mean "*my true
identity.*" My vision went from being just a vision to a compelling
vision. I became compelled to deliver this vision because of the clarity
that I now had. I wrote down the *Adoniaa* vision in my journal:

I felt so good that day with the newfound knowledge that God
gave me concerning my business that I started to call it a Kingdom

Business. The revelation convinced me that I was on a mission for God to empower women to advance His kingdom and, most importantly, create an atmosphere for Him to reign.

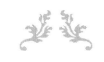

Meanwhile, lipsticks are our flagship products, so my mind went straight to the *Adoniaa* lipsticks that we had given

Our vision is to be a globally respected, one-stop beauty destination helping women at different life stages to connect to their authentic, individual, and unique beauty.

Adedoyin Omotara

mainstream lipstick names before my divine encounter with the Holy Spirit. Lipstick names such as Scandalous, Ruby-red, Spell-bound, Dangerous, etc., I mean those were the kind of names lipsticks in the mainstream beauty world had, so I named mine that way too. I smiled at my foolishness in trying to do what was trending when I could get a blueprint from God. I was even more thankful for how God shed light on my business with this encounter.

After this encounter, the questions I was asking myself changed completely to '*Who must I become to deliver this vision?*' I started to see myself in a different light. I realized that I was not my career or job. Neither was I all the other roles I played as a daughter, wife, mom, or friend. My job, marriage, children, family, and friends were part of the wealth God had given me to deliver His assignment for me successfully.

Introduction

I started reading books that other visionaries had written, began to align myself with the right communities, and generally became more deliberate about how I wanted to live my life, knowing and understanding the vision ahead of me. I started to identify some of my gifts, like speaking, writing, mentoring, coaching, etc. and began to work on them to improve myself.

The answers to the initial questions I asked myself became more apparent as I became more deliberate in committing my ways to God. He started renewing my identity and made me understand that my identity is revealed in how He sees me, and I should fully embrace that. I began to internalize all those powerful words that He downloaded to me and started preparing myself for the task ahead to help other women embrace their identity in God.

This revelation is the story of how God birthed the vision of *Adoniaa Beauty* through me, which I have entirely embraced because I am the *Adoniaa woman*. He gave me a blueprint to follow, which I am still running with as I stay connected to Him daily to unravel the vision's next steps. I knew it was a big assignment when I started my journey of becoming a woman that would help liberate other women from their identity issues. I first had to become the *Adoniaa woman* to be able to free other *Adoniaa women*.

Since I received this vision, life has more meaning, and I have never gone back to that state of disengagement again, even when there are challenges; there is so much fulfillment and meaning to my life now.

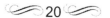

Introduction

I frequently go through the process of rebirthing and becoming to reveal a newer me. I have seen the need to reorganize my life to serve this purpose, cultivate new habits, grow and align myself with the right communities to become the woman who would deliver this vision. This vision birthed everything we do in *Adoniaa Beauty*, Our Marketing strategy, Sales strategy, Campaign strategies, the *"Unmask Your Beauty"* series, *"Unmask Your Beauty"* short films. The *"Unmask Your Beauty"* conferences, Teen Beauty camp, and Women's Beauty camp. This vision birthed this book you are reading right now and many more things that are yet to be unraveled.

It has been four years since the inauguration and launch of *Adoniaa* in Canada, and I have not looked back. I have not had to look back at my plan B to look for a job if my business did not work out because God gave me the vision to run. I have also begun to receive ideas around other areas of my life, and my life keeps evolving.

Dear Adoniaa Woman

I passionately believe that if you make yourself available, God is ready to birth a compelling vision through you because you are His child, and you have complete access to Him. He is waiting for you to embrace and tap into His infinite wisdom for every area of your life

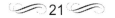

so that you can make use of all the gifts He has deposited inside you to ultimately prepare an atmosphere for Him right here on earth.

The Journey of Transformation

From my transformation journey, I realize that I am not the same woman I was four years ago when God gave me the vision of *Adoniaa Beauty*. I have evolved, and I continue to grow daily into the new woman, now manifesting the vision. This process has taught me that the woman who received the vision is not the same woman who embodies the vision. The woman who embodies the vision is more than ten times the woman who received the vision because she must continually undergo a transformational process to become the woman who manifests the vision.

A more fabulous version of you needs to show up to match the vision God has given to you. The good news is that you have everything it takes to become that woman. You and many others are why I have written this book; to help visionary women like you on your transformational journey to capture a vision and become the woman that delivers it.

You may be in the same place I used to be, where you are confused with life, or you have a vision but do not know how to execute it. This book is designed to help you embrace your true identity, so you can be the woman who houses and manifests the vision God is placing in her heart.

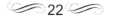

Introduction

In her book *A Return to Love*, author Marianne Williamson said, *"Our deepest fear is not that we are inadequate. Our deepest fear is that we are powerful beyond measure. It is our light, not our darkness that most frightens us. We ask ourselves, 'Who am I to be brilliant, gorgeous, talented, fabulous?' Who are you not to be? You are a child of God. Playing it safe does not serve the world. There is nothing enlightened about shrinking so that other people will not feel insecure around you. We are all meant to shine as children do. We were born to make manifest the glory of God that is within us. It is not just in some of us; it is in everyone. And as we let our light shine, we unconsciously permit other people to do the same. As we are liberated from our fear, our presence automatically liberates others."*

Dear Adoniaa Woman

As you read this book, the world is waiting for your manifestation because you are the solution someone is waiting for, so get yourself ready to become the woman that delivers. You are beautiful, valuable, worthy of every good thing, and powerful beyond measure no matter what your background, past experiences, and society have made you believe that you are. Let go of all labels, shame, guilt, hurt, and fear that has been masking your beauty. Go out there and unmask all the beauty that you hold within!

Introduction

In the following chapters, I will be taking you through a 4-stage process to help you unmask all the beauty that you hold inside you so you can become the woman that delivers the vision God has placed in her heart. These are stages God alone takes us through; our role is to be present and participate through surrender.

Transformation simply means closing the gap between where you are and where you are going. The different transformational stages refer to the different stages a woman could be at in her evolutionary journey to a life of meaning and success. We may find parts of these different phases expressed in our lives simultaneously, but we usually find one stage which speaks the most to where we are. Women can also go back and forth along these stages at different seasons of life.

To best understand how these four stages unfold, think of them as the stages of pregnancy. Knowing that a baby is coming gives you greater confidence, clarity, readiness, and resilience. It helps you understand what to prepare for and what to expect when you are expecting.

The process of personal transformation works the same way; only no one ever describes how the process takes place - what battles you will face, what feelings and doubts you will encounter, or what you can do to enjoy and thrive through the process. If you know a baby is coming and that labor pains, cravings, and mood swings are part of the process, you are likely to be more resilient and able to press through. The abnormal becomes normal - tears, hormonal changes, and weight

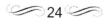

gain come with the territory. But you would not know that if you had never experienced it or if no one ever explained it.

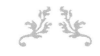

That is my mission with the *"Unmask Your Beauty"* book. I do not want you to get stuck in the past, in betrayal, regret, self-doubt, or even something as positive as your last success. I want you to maximize your life, fully unleashing what

To write a great book, you must first become the book.

Adedoyin Omotara

God has in you because He needs you, I need you, and others need what God has exclusively placed within you to birth. I intend to walk beside you and help you gain greater clarity about what you've been through, what you will go through, and what God has in store for you as long as you keep pressing through. It is also my mission to help you tap into and *"Unmask Your Beauty"* by embracing the higher version of you that is seeking to emerge right now.

The stages I describe in this book are all stages I have gone through myself and am still going through because unmasking is a continuous transformation process where you are continually birthing newer versions of yourself.

To drive home some of my points in this book, I have shared some of my personal stories and shared real *Adoniaa women's* personal stories, but I have changed some names to protect their privacy.

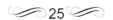

Introduction

Get ready for a transformational journey into revealing the hidden truth of who you are indeed in the eyes of God.

Adedoyin

For maximum benefit,
I encourage you to get a journal
to gather all your thoughts down on paper.

Stage 1 - AWAKEN

Your Current Life Assessment
Identifying Masks
The Process of Unmasking

Every transformational journey starts with an awakening. To awaken means to observe our behavior and to align ourselves with the truth. A genuine awakening causes you to recognize that much of what you previously thought or understood was quite limited or partial. The awakening is a process involving many types of awareness and painful confrontations. Hard work for sure, but in the end, nothing could be more valuable or worthwhile. For me, I was awakened by the dissatisfaction I felt in my career. I believed I had so much more within me and realized that I lived by societal standards for success and significance until I decided to create a life true to who God says I am. Your story may be different; it could be your finances, your relationships, your health, or other areas of your life that will birth this awakening into a more incredible version of you.

My question for you is: In what area of your life are you currently going through dissatisfaction, and you know that it does not align with who you truly are or who you desire to become? The good news is that you have the power to turn things around.

01 Your Current Life Assessment

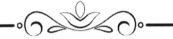

In this step, we will start by assessing the current state of your life. Before renovating a building, regardless of how detailed the blueprint may be, the builder must first inspect the building's current condition.

View this assessment as looking into each room in your life. If we are going to be renovating your home, we need to peek into each room and see what needs the most attention right now. You want to be as authentic as possible. Your journal is for you alone, so feel free to pour out your heart into it. Put all your thoughts down on paper and write as much as you can.

Health

Mind

- ☐ Do you have a positive outlook on life?
- ☐ Do you struggle with depression or anxiety? If so, have you seen a doctor?
- ☐ How do you deal with daily stresses?
- ☐ How do you handle sudden, overwhelming stress such as loss of a job, home, etc.?
- ☐ Do you believe you are capable of change?

Body

- ☐ How do you sleep?
- ☐ What are your eating habits like?
- ☐ Do you maintain a healthy diet?
- ☐ What is your overall perception of your body?
- ☐ Do you exercise regularly?
- ☐ Do you go for your yearly medical checkup? If so, do you follow your doctor's advice?
- ☐ Are you dealing with any addictions, diseases, or chronic conditions? Have you sought professional care where needed?

Spirit

- How do you define spirituality? Do you consider yourself a spiritual person?
- What are you doing to feed and inspire your spirit? If you are not doing anything, why not?
- Do you feel a sense of purpose in your life? Something more significant than you. Explain.

Self-image

Self-esteem

- When you walk out the door every day, what do you feel?
- How do you feel about your appearance and wardrobe selections?
- Are you accurately representing who you are?
- Do you speak up for yourself when needed?

Attitude

- Do you feel like your outlook is positive or negative?
- How does your attitude affect your work and relationships?
- How would others describe your attitude?

Appearance

- When you look in the mirror, do you feel beautiful?

- Do you feel you have an authentic style?
- What is your greatest need right now? Hair, makeup, wardrobe, something else?
- How do you think you are perceived when others meet you?

Relationships

Romance

- Are you single or in a relationship?
- Are you happy with your current relationship status?
- If you are in a relationship, do you feel supported and valued?
- Do you have a bond of unconditional love?
- Are you able to be completely honest and open with your partner?
- Do you find ways to keep the romance alive?
- Do you give time and energy every week to expressing love in your life (toward yourself and others)?

Friendship

- Do you feel invigorated or drained after spending time with your friends?
- Do your friends love and support you unconditionally?
- How often do you spend time with your friends?

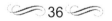

Are you able to be completely honest and open with your friends?

Family

How would you describe your relationship with your immediate family and with your extended family?

Do you support and love each other unconditionally? Why or why not?

Do you spend quality time together every week? If not, what can you do to increase the amount or quality of the time you do spend together?

Career

Current Job

Do you love your job?

If yes, what do you love about your job?

What would you change about your job if you could?

Goals

How do you define success?

Do you consider yourself successful? If not, what is holding you back?

What are your career goals? Are you on track to achieving these goals?

Finances

Current Spending Habits

- ☐ Do you have a budget? Why or why not?
- ☐ Do you live within this budget (if you have one)?

- ☐ Are you able to live comfortably?
- ☐ Are you in control of your spending habits?

Future Needs & Retirement

- ☐ Are you financially stable?
- ☐ Are you able to save and invest money?
- ☐ Do you have a financial plan for your future?
- ☐ Are you on track to meeting your retirement needs?

How does it feel to get your current life situation on paper? This exercise is immensely powerful and will help you understand where you are in different areas of your life. I am sure that you are incredibly happy with some areas of your life, while you probably desire to improve some other parts of your life. However, there may also be some areas you are not satisfied with at all, and you believe there is more for you. Something in you tells you that this is not all there is to you. You know that you are not aligning with who you are at your core. The good news is that you have the power to deliberately change every area of your life to get the results that match your identity in God.

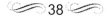

The first time I did my life assessment, I was already in the middle of changing careers from project management in the oil and gas industry into entrepreneurship in the beauty industry. I wanted to explore entrepreneurship after I had spent eight years in IT & project management. I was able to get to the root of why I kept doing jobs that did not give me fulfillment but conformed to what society expected of me. I had seen this modeled by everyone around me, so I automatically thought I had to do the same.

I traced back the root of developing a great sense of confidence in myself to things I saw modeled by my parents when I was in Grade 4. There were only eight students in my class, and five were school prefects. A prefect is a student who has been identified as a leader and given specific school responsibilities. I felt so disappointed that I was not one of the five chosen. I thought that I deserved to be a school prefect, given my academic records and my comportment in class. I immediately felt that I had no worth.

I went home crying and told my dad what had happened. He said I should not care about what anyone thought I could do or not do. He told me, *"Doyin, you are very responsible. I admire the way you look after your younger siblings. You are brilliant. You are very proactive."* After my dad highlighted all my strengths, I felt good and no longer cared that I was not a prefect at school; after all, I was a prefect in my head.

That was one of the incidents that I remember shaping my thinking early in my life. My dad practically brainwashed me into believing that even if other people thought that I was not the most qualified person for something, I should still believe that I was the woman for the job, as long as I desired it. *"Thank you, daddy!"*

Dear Adoniaa Woman

Whatever results you are currently getting in your life reflect your state of mind and how you are thinking. If you are not happy with your current results, you need to get to the root cause of that thinking or mindset. We often try to change our outcome like it is something external. What we do not know is that we must do the internal work first. We must fix the programming for new developments to begin to show in our lives.

In the next chapter, I will help you get to the root of the thinking and mindset that created your current life assessment realities. We will be focusing on the parts of your life that are misaligned with who you want to be. We will also begin to identify the masks stopping you from being your best self in those areas of your life.

02: Identifying Masks

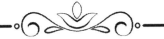

We often unconsciously wear masks that prevent us from becoming our best selves and manifesting all that God has created us to do. A considerable part of awakening is identifying those masks and consciously trying to unmask. We were not born with masks; we mask ourselves based on what we saw modeled for us in childhood or other life experiences. The masks we wear generally reflect what the society or culture around us promotes, but we have the power to take off these masks.

We can identify masks in different areas of our lives if we decide to be true to ourselves. However, identifying these masks can be challenging as different areas of our lives may be hidden by multiple masks.

As mentioned earlier, I worked in the corporate world for eight years because of what I believed about having a career modeled by my parents.

I believed that my career was my identity, and the more money I had, the more people would respect me. I saw a lot of that while growing up. People would gather in my parents' house asking for money or different types of favors. My dad had a great career and was well respected. He also helped a lot of family and friends to establish themselves. I believed I had to have a corporate career and rise to the top of my career just like him. Deep down, I felt that if I lost my job, the people around me would see me as a failure, and I would lose my identity. So, I kept getting additional training and certifications and changing jobs and roles to prove a point to myself. I went for more challenging positions to be respected and feel better about myself until I started to feel uncomfortable and resolved to see myself in a different light. I now choose to view myself as God sees me, regardless of the work that I do.

The transition into entrepreneurship also came with its own masks. The *Adoniaa Beauty* product line launch brought an overwhelming feeling of fear and rejection. I was also suffering from impostor syndrome. According to Wikipedia, impostor syndrome is a psychological pattern in which one doubts one's accomplishments and has a persistent internalized fear of being exposed as a fraud. I felt like a fraud because I believed that people like me did not create and launch

products for different skin types. As I was
not living in my country of origin, I thought
no one would accept my products in
Canada because of my skin color. Who was
I to create a diverse shade of beauty
products for women of all shades and skin
types? I did not look like the type of people
who succeeded with a beauty product line
in a place like Canada. I felt the likes of

Masks can distort
our identity.

Adedoyin Omotara

Mary Kay, Bobbi Brown were better than me, and the beauty industry
was not for me. I tried to go to women events that were full of white
people just to seek approval, but in the end, none of those things helped,
until I started to see myself as God saw me, and He began to show me
the blueprint of how to do Kingdom work. Now *Adoniaa Beauty* has a
diverse clientele base, which has completely embraced our brand.

From my career stories, I identified fear of failure, fear of
rejection, low self-esteem, and impostor syndrome as masks I was
wearing that did not let my real beauty shine through and hindered me
from becoming all that God had in store for me.

Masks can distort our identity, so we need to be very aware to
accurately identify our masks and get into the habit of unmasking to
become our best selves.

From my personal experience and working with numerous
women, I have learned that women who wear masks hide behind hidden

emotions. These emotions range from fear of failure, rejection, guilt, shame, depression, low self-esteem, self-doubt, addiction, feelings of worthlessness, impostor syndrome, bitterness, self-sabotage, unforgiveness, resentment, and more.

The above emotions often represent masks in our lives, making us feel unworthy, condemned, and prevent us from embracing who we indeed are. We wear different types of masks at various stages of our lives based on how our minds have been conditioned to think, so we need to intentionally recondition our minds toward who God says we are.

Our current reality reflects our beliefs about who we are. It is usually consistent with what we think to be true about ourselves. Our feelings, behaviors, and views all interact to shape our lives.

I have outlined some of the false or limiting belief systems I have identified in women below, along with how they show up and the masks they come in.

False Belief System	Symptom	Emotions /Masks
I must meet specific standards to attain self-worth and feel good about myself.	Perfectionism Unhealthy drive to succeed	Fear of failure

False Belief System	Symptom	Emotions /Masks
I am not good enough, or I am not deserving of some good things in life.	Attempt to please others. Being overly sensitive to criticism Withdrawal from others to avoid disapproval	Fear of rejection Low self-esteem Impostor syndrome
I have failed before, so I will not try again. What if I fail again? (past failures)	Blaming of self and others for personal failure Withdrawal from God and people	Fear of failure Fear of punishment
What you see is who I am, I cannot change (e.g., I am not good with money, I am not good with people) - generally holding on to labels.	Repeated patterns of behavior	Feelings of shame Hopelessness Inferiority, Passivity Loss of creativity Isolation or withdrawal from others Depression

From the table, I am sure you can identify with one or more belief systems, symptoms, and masks. This list is not exhaustive, and you may be dealing with other types of belief systems, so please feel free to add yours.

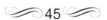

The bondage of masks and belief systems is often deeply rooted in our personalities, patterns of behavior, and ways of relating to other people. The specific effects of false belief systems and resulting actions vary from person to person, depending on family background, personality traits, culture, relationships, and many other factors.

The Roots of Our Belief System

I believe that all these false belief systems have roots, and to unmask fully, we need to trace them down to their roots. Your roots may be different from mine as we all have different backgrounds, grew up in different environments, and have different childhood and life experiences.

Identifying the roots of your belief system is especially vital to your unmasking completely and becoming a more credible version of yourself.

The root of most of our belief systems is generated from a concept called 'subconscious conditioning.'

The subconscious is the part of your mind that operates below your average level of waking consciousness. It is like the operating system of your mind, so we need to be very deliberate about what goes in there. Right now, you are primarily using your conscious mind to read these words and absorb their meaning. Still, beneath that mental focus, your subconscious mind is busily working behind the scenes, absorbing or rejecting information based on an existing perception of the world around you. This current perception began forming when you were an infant.

With every experience, your subconscious mind soaks in information like a sponge. It rejected nothing while you were young because you did not have any pre-existing beliefs to filter what it received. It only accepted that all the information you received during your early childhood was accurate. You can probably see why this becomes a problem later in life. Whenever someone called you stupid, worthless, slow, lazy, or worse as a child, your subconscious mind just stored the information away for future reference. You may also have received messages about your potential in life or limitations you will face based on your physical abilities, skin color, gender, or economic status. Now that you are an adult, you may think you can simply discard the hurtful or untrue messages you absorbed during your early life, but it is not quite that simple.

Remember that all this information is stored below your level of conscious awareness. The only time you become aware of it is when it limits your progress in creating a balanced, successful, and productive life, just like when I became aware that society and my environment had defined my career for me.

Napoleon Hill wrote in his book *Think and Grow Rich:* *"Your subconscious mind does not reason; it does not analyze nor think. It just does what it has been trained to do by its master, YOU and ME! If I plant a lot of weeds in my garden, I will get loads of weeds but if I plant*

*loads of organic vegetables, guess what, I will get loads of great organic
vegetables! It won't judge or help you if you didn't want weeds; you just
reap what you sow."*

Our thoughts and actions have been stored and memorized in
such a way to keep us within our comfort zone. If we let this happen to
us and we do not sow the right seeds in our minds, not only will we get
garbage, but that garbage will make things even worse and reinforce
what has happened in our past, which will most likely produce more of
that negative thinking!

So, if there are any areas of your life where you have ever tried
to achieve a goal and kept sabotaging yourself at every turn, it is
essential to know that you are not defective or doomed to fail. More than
likely, you have got some old, programmed messages in your
subconscious mind that conflict with the new conditions you want to
create.

This revelation about the mind is excellent news because it
means you can achieve just about anything if you take the time to
reprogram your subconscious mind.

First, let us identify some of the roots of the belief systems that
we have, which have resulted in creating masks in our lives.

The Root of Childhood Experiences

Our childhood experiences have a significant influence on who
we are today at the deepest level. Our environment shaped many of our

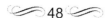

beliefs while growing up based on what was modeled to us by our parents, caregivers, family members, culture, and society.

If we take the time to reflect on how much of what we do and think did not originate as God's idea for us and let go of things that do not serve us; we will be free to embrace beliefs and life choices that genuinely resonate with who God says we are and live the life we were truly born to live. We need to peel away the layers of belief systems that do not serve who God says we are. Removing these masks may be challenging because even though they hold us back from our true selves, they provide a sense of comfort.

To break a belief system, it is essential to keep in mind our reasons for changing that way of thinking. By imagining living our lives as who God says we are, we begin creating a different reality that will grow and blossom with time.

Meet Adoniaa Woman, Ronny

Her family neglected Ronny as a child, and because of this, other students constantly bullied Ronny at school, which gradually started affecting her sense of worth. Based on what she saw around her, she became a bully herself, hung out with bad gangs, and became homeless. She later moved in with her drug-dealer boyfriend at age sixteen, who beat her until she landed in the emergency department. This experience led to an awakening for her, and she started to consider a better life. Something in her told her that there had to be more to life. Her current position could not be the best life. Ronny played out her childhood experiences into her teenage years until she discovered that way of life did not align with the core of who she was. She saw that she could do better with herself and rewrite her story going forward despite all her childhood traumas. Ronny sought help and started to recondition her mind. Now, she uses her story as a message to empower other young people to align with who God says they are.

Meet Adoniaa Woman, Lois

Lois grew up in a very abusive home and was molested by her father repeatedly. She grew up feeling completely worthless, and her mind had been conditioned not to value herself. Lois started to trade her body for money. One day, she found out that one of the men she had gone to a brothel with was a serial killer. That was her awakening moment because she felt he could have killed her, but God rescued her. Lois started to see herself differently and began making changes by volunteering with companies that championed causes that mattered to her. She began to visualize a better life for herself and began to recover from her addictions by coming to terms with who she currently was and who she was becoming. Now, Lois is employing her neighbors and taking people off the streets and training them to work for her cleaning company. She also speaks to inspire people to dream bigger and wake up to the light.

The Root of Environmental /Societal /Cultural Conditioning

Some belief systems that we have internalized as women have distorted our sense of identity. These systems came about when we were young girls observing our environment, culture, and society at large. For example, as women, we have specific belief systems around the following:

1) Marriage

As women, culture, and society have told us that we must get married to live a meaningful life. We were programmed to search for our Prince Charming. Physical beauty then becomes a priority, and we soon learn that is also who and what Prince Charming wants. Once we get married, many of us think our identity and sufficiency is in being a wife and having a successful marriage that others admire and emulate. Marriage can be fantastic if you marry and find the best man for you. However, your marriage is not who you are. It is not your identity. Family studies have shown that women are generally happier in marriage when they bring their unique identity into their marriages and are not trying to hide under their husbands' shadow or the institution of marriage.

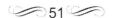

Meet Adoniaa Woman, Bella

Bella's mother was a happy homemaker married to her successful father. As she grew up, Bella dreamt of having the life modeled by her parents. She lived her mom's life for the first 12 years of her marriage until she finally realized that her identity did not come from her husband's successes or her marriage. Bella reached out to me, and we got to the root of what made her think that was the sum of her life. She identified that she was living her mom's life because her mom was happy and had unconsciously defined success for her. Bella saw that she had tied her identity to her husband's accomplishments and could not even answer the question— *"Who am I?"* We started to work together on understanding her identity, and she is now able to bring more value to her marriage with the discoveries she is making about herself.

2) Motherhood

As young girls, we were taught that as women, we must bear children of our own, and as soon as we start having children, we begin to see motherhood as our identity. We begin to attach our identity to our children. Even if you do not have children, you might believe that part of your identity as a woman means having children and celebrating it. Being a mother is a gift from God and part of the wealth God has given you, but it is not your identity. It is not who you are.

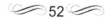

Meet *Adoniaa Woman, Becky*

Becky turned 40, and suddenly she began to feel uneasy within herself. She began to ask herself what she had spent the last 40 years of her life doing? Becky realized that her main dreams in life were to get married and have children. She had spent the first 30 years of her life finding a good man to marry and the next ten years raising her children. Suddenly, Becky started feeling disengaged with life even though she had a happy family. Becky soon realized that her life not only consisted of marriage and kids; however, this mindset had been promoted by her mom and aunties, so she unconsciously relived the experiences of the women who had raised her. Once she realized this, she started connecting with the truth of who she was and began to dream again.

3) Career

When your identity is tied to work, career, and building a professional or business legacy. We find our value and worth in our work, the titles we earn, the checks we make, the clothes we wear, the offices we hold, the awards we win, the perceived impact we have, and how impressive we look. When people ask us who we are. We say we are doctors, engineers, nurses, lawyers, entrepreneurs, etc.

Identifying Masks

Dear Adoniaa Woman

You are not your career or job. Your job or career is a platform God has given you to influence and serve people by living in your true God-given identity as a child of God.

Meet Adoniaa Woman, Tawnya

Tawnya grew up with extraordinarily successful parents. Her parents were both engineers. Her parents' successes modeled to her as she was growing up made her believe this was the only way for her to succeed. Tawnya ended up working for a multinational oil and gas company as an engineer. After working there for several years, she later realized that she was not happy with the job, and the job did not bring out the best in her. It was difficult to leave this belief system behind, where Tawnya attached her self-worth to her career. Her career had built a comfortable life for her that made her parents proud, but she was also an artistic person, highly creative, and good with her hands. After realizing that the root of her belief system was not true to her, she started to focus on the things she truly desired based on her strengths and passions, and now she is on her way to building a life of her dreams.

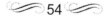

The Root of Life Experiences

Life experiences can alter your belief systems even as an adult and not just as a child. Some people base their reality on what they have been through in life. You may have gone through some life experiences that have shaped you into who you are today. Your experience could be a divorce or the loss of a loved one. Another experience could be emotional, physical, or sexual abuse. It could also be repeated patterns of failure that may have made you believe that you are not good enough. These feelings could make you withdraw from people, become resentful, or even self-harm. God does not want you to see yourself in the light of these experiences. God wants you to see yourself as He sees you despite the things the enemy throws at you.

Meet Adoniaa Woman, Shona

At the age of 50, Shona went through an ugly separation after 30 years of an emotionally abusive marriage that she had sacrificed her career and many other things for. During that period of separation, she lost her daughter, who had suffered a protracted illness. Notwithstanding, her husband pressed forward with the divorce so that he could settle down with his mistress.

Shona contemplated suicide to end it all as an option as she was feeling very worthless, isolated, and was suffering from Major Depressive Disorder with features of anxiety.

At about this time, she was introduced to a local church by a friend. The church leadership identified her vulnerability, closely followed up with her, and became her primary support. They helped her start a new life by reconditioning her mind with scriptures that helped her heal. She formed new relationships and consolidated existing ones. The divorce led Shona to a period of awakening. Shona suddenly realized that she was not any of the labels she had identified as in the past. She started to believe the truth about who God said she was and started to dream again.

Today, 20 years post-divorce, she is happy that she did not commit suicide. The rest of her family and friends are so proud of her as she has become a strong pillar of support for people going through similar hard times, helping them identify the positives in their lives and letting them know that they can have a new beginning.

Identifying Masks

Dear Adoniaa Woman

Whenever you wake up is your morning, I am sure some of the stories I have shared resonate with you, and even if they do not, you can plug in your own story and start to get to the root of the emotions masking your true beauty, which is your true identity in God. I hope that my story and the stories of other Adoniaa women in this book will inspire you to start to create a life that is true to God's desires for your life.

Exercise:

This exercise is powerful, and it is the start of your journey into unmasking. Based on your life assessment in Step 1 of the Awaken Stage, identify the areas of your life you are dissatisfied with:

- The areas where you believe that there is more inside you, and you can do better.
- Identify the belief systems that are not serving you.
- Trace the belief system down to the different root causes identified in Stage 2.
- Write down the story of the event that created the belief system.
- Write down the symptom you are currently exhibiting and the emotions or masks that come with that symptom.

For each mask, ask yourself these questions,

- Where did you learn to wear the mask?
- Who told you (or modeled) how to wear the mask?
- How would you like your life to look for you to feel that you are living in alignment with your true self?
- Is there anyone affected by you letting go of the masks that do not serve you?
- What benefit do you get from maintaining these masks the way they are?
- What benefits would you get from removing your masks?

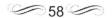

- Who would you become if the masks you do not want any more were to disappear?

Area of life that I am not satisfied with	False belief system	Roots of belief system	Story of the incident that created the false belief system	Symptom	Emotions /masks

03: The Process of Unmasking

Now that you have identified your masks, the belief systems creating the masks, and the roots of your belief systems, you can start the process of unmasking.

How do you unmask? You unmask by moving closer to who God wants you to be. Focus your energy not on the masks themselves but by looking to the other side where you believe God wants you to be. The unmasking process to uncover the real you begins with eliminating belief systems that do not serve you by reprogramming your mind.

Reprogramming your mind is taking active control of your mind and redirecting your focus to making your life a masterpiece. Your mind is the key to success, and you have the power to learn how to reprogram your subconscious. There is no better time to take back control of your mind and set your sights on something better than right now.

When I was 13 years old, my dad married a second wife. My mom, myself, and all my siblings felt so disappointed, let down, and hurt—my dad's actions filled my world with many negative emotions. I felt so ashamed that I did not even tell my best friend, Fehintoluwa, for three years, until it finally settled in my mind that this was the new normal for us. I did not see it coming because we were close to our dad and just could not imagine it. This event changed everything for me, and I hid it from many of my friends in school because I felt that people would judge and mistreat me if they knew that I was from a polygamous home. At some point, I started to think I was not deserving of good things, which began to affect my studies. I remember just wishing I could blank out that part of my life. My mom was utterly dehumanized, and we were all angry.

As we began to vent our anger, we started withdrawing from our dad, who had been our best friend until then. The company our dad worked for transferred him to Abuja, so he relocated with his new wife and came to visit us occasionally in Ibadan. Later he wanted us to spend our holidays with him in Abuja, which we rejected because of how he had treated us.

After a few years, my dad called my mom, siblings, and I into a room and apologized immensely. He said he was deeply sorry for what his actions had caused us and that he loved us very much and did not want to alienate us. He cried and said he was deeply sorry. That melted our hearts, and that was how we all began the journey of forgiving him.

I decided to forgive my dad, we all did, and our relationship started to thrive again. We decided to embrace each other as a family, and I am now proud of our mega-size happy family. I now proudly tell people that I have six sisters and one brother. I am forever thankful for the gift of friendship that I have with all my siblings, never a dull moment.

However, my mind became conditioned by what my dad had done. I vowed never to get emotionally attached to any man, so I would not be hurt if he cheated on me. As a woman, I also decided that I would always be financially empowered, so I would not need to depend on any man to meet my financial needs. You see the way the mind works? That was what I saw as a child, and that was how I interpreted the situation.

As a result of this conditioning, I became overly sensitive to anything that affected a woman's rights. I remember standing up for one of my high school friends because the boys had given her a defamatory award at the students' awards night. The students' awards night was supposed to be a fun night at the end of the school year organized by students living in the hostel. My friend was given an award called the Cowbell Award, simply because, according to the boys, she had big breasts. I found it so defamatory that I carefully planned out how to retaliate at the next award season with seven of my girlfriends. Of course, we went too far with it and ended up in trouble, but I was happy.

That was the only way I could fight for her and not allow the boys to get away with humiliating her.

As I started evolving and becoming a young woman, my mindset about men gradually changed when I started seeing many beautiful marriages that I admired. I lived with one of my mom's best friends while I was at university, and I saw her and her husband model a marriage based on trust and love, so my beliefs about marriage gradually began to change. Also, I had to tell myself that it was not my fault that my dad married a second wife. I began to detach myself completely from the identity that said *"I come from a polygamous home, so I am not good enough,"* to *"I am a child of God, and I can make choices that will create a new path for me."*

I started visualizing a lot about what I wanted for my future, especially in my marriage. I am thankful that I did not allow my own childhood experiences to condition my mind about my amazing husband, who I fondly call Babyluv.

Based on my own experiences and the experiences of hundreds of women who have shared their stories with me, I have identified six ways to reprogram our mind as we embark on the journey of unmasking to reveal our best selves.

#1 Forgive

Forgiveness is simply a deliberate decision to release feelings of resentment or vengeance you have toward a person who has harmed you, regardless of whether they deserve your forgiveness or not. One does not have to return to the same relationship with an offender or accept the offender's harmful behavior. Forgiveness is a decision you need to make, most especially for your mental health. Not forgiving someone means you are holding on to painful emotions, and unforgiveness will cause you

> When you change your self-talk, you change your world.
>
> Adedoyin Omotara

more negativity than the person you are not forgiving, so forgiving others is really for you because it frees you of negative emotions.

#2 Adopt Empowering Beliefs

False or limiting beliefs hold us back from what we want in life. Some people's false beliefs are based on their past results, adverse events they have experienced, or a flawed vision of their future. When you address these beliefs and challenge their accuracy, you can replace them with empowering beliefs. From my story, it would be replacing, *"I am from a polygamous family, so I do not deserve the best relationships,"* to *"I deserve the best relationship with someone I truly love because I am deserving of every good thing."* When you change your self-talk, you change your world.

#3 Focus on Gratitude

When you choose gratitude and appreciation over criticism and fear, you shine a light on the positive. This choice rewires your brain to notice more of what you have and less of what you don't have. It also allows you to be curious about the events in your life as you no longer view them with suspicion. You can embrace change and let it in, appreciating that life never stays the same. My mom gradually healed from the hurt caused by my dad by focusing on gratitude and prayers. To date, I attribute all our successes in life to my mom's attitude of gratitude and her prayers. Her attitude of gratitude is so contagious that we, her children, also decided to focus on gratitude. We stopped focusing on *"our dad has a second wife"* and shifted our focus to *"Our dad still cares about us and takes care of us"* because we had seen situations where the husband disowned the first wife and children. Gratitude is not about condoning hurtful behavior, but it helps you recondition your mind so that you only focus on what is serving you, and by doing so, you will attract more of it and start to dream again.

#4 Align Yourself with the Right Communities

When reprogramming your brain for success, you must limit negative influences in your environment. Your subconscious mind is constantly absorbing information from external sources and using that information to form beliefs that shape how you think and behave.

Negativity from the daily news, toxic people, and social media can profoundly affect your subconscious mind without you even knowing it.

As you work on how to reprogram your mind, remember that proximity is power. Surround yourself with positive, supportive people. Seek out books, videos, and music that uplift and empower you. Over time, you will find that your subconscious mind is more positive and encouraging and that negative thoughts have greatly diminished.

#5 Visualize

Your subconscious mind responds well to pictures. Visualization is a great way to program your mind with positive, empowering images. Try spending 10–15 minutes a day visualizing positive scenes that feature you and your life experiences. Here are some things you may want to visualize:

- Fulfilling relationships
- Passionate work
- A beautiful home
- Anything else you wish to draw into your life

As you do this consistently, you will eventually replace the negative pictures from your past experiences, fears, worries, and doubts with images of a better future. To further boost the power of visualization, be sure to emit strong, positive emotions while you imagine these beautiful things in your mind. Allow feelings of love, joy, gratitude, and peace to flow through you as if you are genuinely having these experiences. Your subconscious mind will absorb the messages as if they are real! This is the true beauty of visualization - the power to bypass limiting messages and focus on pleasing images, all of which are being absorbed right into your subconscious to be replayed later.

#6 Affirmations

Affirmations are another effective way to install positive messages into your subconscious. They work best if you follow a few simple rules:

Word them positively and in the present tense. Say *"I am confident and successful"* rather than *"I will be confident and successful"* because focusing on a future condition does not compute with your subconscious mind—it only knows this moment.

Call up the corresponding feelings. Saying *"I am wealthy"* while feeling poor only sends conflicting messages to your subconscious. Whatever words you say, strive to feel the corresponding emotions, then your subconscious will be more likely to believe it.

Repeat, repeat, repeat. Affirmations do not work if you say them just once or twice. For best results, recite them many times throughout the day. The good thing is that you can fit your affirmations seamlessly into your daily routine since you can say them to yourself whenever you choose to.

Exercise:

1. Using your responses from your life assessment (Step 1 of the Awaken Stage) and the masks identified (in Step 2), list the emotions you need to start unmasking.

2. Start the process of forgiving the people who have hurt you by doing the following:

   - Decide to forgive them.
   - Write out the names of the people you need to forgive.
   - Write out what you forgive them.
   - Write out all the emotions you are still feeling.
   - Write - *I forgive you.*
   - Burn or shred the paper - This is to put action to what you have decided to do. It is a powerful exercise.
   - Write down five ways you plan to *"Unmask Your Beauty"* daily.

Stage 1 Summary:

How are you feeling right now after doing the exercises? Feel free to let out all your emotions in your journal. I applaud you for beginning the process of identifying your masks and removing them, which is an excellent start to the life that God genuinely wants for you. Now that you have started to recondition your mind to what is possible in your life, the next stage is to discover yourself so you can step into your

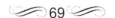

power. For any significant shift to occur, you need to understand who you are and how to leverage your power.

Stage 2 - DISCOVER YOURSELF

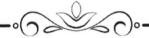

Who Are You?
You Are Uniquely Wired
Why Are You Here?

I began to pay more attention to myself when I left my job and started building *Adoniaa Beauty* because I knew that the decisions I made, my choices, and responses to challenges, and generally, every input into *Adoniaa* would flow out of me. So, I needed to understand who I was at my core, how I was naturally wired, and how I could cultivate and leverage my unique gifts and talents. This never occurred to me when I worked in the corporate world; no wonder I felt so disengaged. Looking back now, I would advise anyone to start self-discovery as early as twelve years old and repeat the exercise yearly. Self-discovery will help ground you and enable you to make the best decisions for your life.

From my experience, the process of discovering yourself is an ongoing progression rather than a static snapshot. You should embrace a flowing sense of self, whereby you are perpetually reframing, reorganizing, rethinking, rebirthing, and unmasking yourself. You have already started the process of unmasking by mastering a daily process of reconditioning your mind to think better thoughts and heal yourself of all the emotions that mask who you are. Now that you are consciously choosing your thoughts, you need to understand what makes you unique, which takes you into self-discovery.

Self-discovery is the process of knowing who you are at your core, identifying the things that make you unique based on how you are innately wired, and embracing the truth about you. This process is not to put you into a box but to make you more aware of everything unique about you so you can leverage it to birth a higher version of yourself.

In this section, I will walk you through a self-discovery process based on who you are, how you are uniquely wired, and why you are here on earth.

04: Who Are You?

Psalm 139:13-16 (NIV)

13 For you created my inmost being;

you knit me together in my mother's womb.

14 I praise you because I am fearfully and wonderfully made;

your works are wonderful,

I know that full well.

15 My frame was not hidden from you

when I was made in the secret place,

when I was woven together in the depths of the earth.

16 Your eyes saw my unformed body;

all the days ordained for me were written in your book

before one of them came to be.

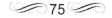

In Stage 1 of this book, we talked about The Awakening. You will agree that every woman's deepest craving is to find a sense of significance or relevance. Unfortunately, we have allowed culture and society to define how we search for significance. That is why we have embraced titles such as having a degree, working in a big company, being someone's wife, and being someone's mom as our identity. We have tried to look for significance in all the wrong places. We look for it through our career, professional accomplishments, educational qualifications, marriage, children, etc. We think that all these labels will make us significant and successful. But no label will ever fill the void of significance and success until we trace our roots back to the one who created us.

In this self-discovery process, the first question I will put to you is, "where are you from?" Because you can never know who you are if you do not know where you came from. If you try to find where you are from based on your earthly heritage, you will lose your way because you can never get a full picture from there. We can only find answers to this question by knowing and connecting with the One who created us

Then God said, "Let us make mankind in our image, in our likeness, so that they may rule over the fish in the sea and the birds in the sky, over the livestock and all the wild animals, and over all the

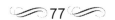

creatures that move along the ground." So, God
created mankind in his own image, in the image of
God he created them; male and female he created
them.

Genesis 1:26-27 (NIV)

The word image jumps out at me from this scripture, and I would love to explore it. According to Online Dictionary, an image is an a physical likeness or representation of a person, animal, or thing, photographed, painted, sculptured, or otherwise made visible.

Like most manufacturers, *Adoniaa's* logo is placed on all our products after they have undergone rigorous testing before being released into circulation. We are assured of the products' success because of the quality of the ingredients they are made from. All of these make us very confident about releasing our product line to the world. *Adoniaa's* product success is my success because it is a brand I created based on my beliefs and values.

Likewise, that is how God created us. He placed His logo on us by making us in His image. He instilled His qualities and everything that He is in us before launching us into the world. We were already finished products, wholly tested before birth. Our success was pre-guaranteed because it is God's success. God wants us to succeed because He has stamped us with His image. Our success in this world is of great value to God, but we keep looking at other places to find it instead of connecting with God, our manufacturer.

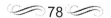

Who Are You?

So, what are these attributes and qualities of God that He has stamped on us? Throughout the scriptures, we see who God is. God is all-powerful, God is love, God is light, God is magnificent, God is strong, God is excellent, God is a creator, etc. God is all these amazing things and more, and guess what? You can be all these and more if only you will believe and completely embody God's image that He has stamped on you.

During my encounter with the Holy Spirit in 2016, this was what God told me to declare to women through *Adoniaa Beauty*. He said I should remind women that He created us in His image.

Dear Adoniaa Woman

I want you to see yourself as God sees you! You are a complete product from God. So, stop looking for yourself in all the wrong places. Your greatest superpower is that you have God's branding, and you have direct access to your manufacturer, God.

God said to Jeremiah in Jeremiah 1:5 (NIV), "Before I formed you in the womb I knew you, before you were born I set you apart; I appointed you as a prophet to the nations."

And in verse 10, He also says,

"See, today I appoint you over nations and kingdoms to uproot and tear down, to destroy and overthrow, to build and to plant."

Who Are You?

God knew you before He even formed you, and He has an excellent plan for you. He loves you so much, and He wants you to realize this and imitate His nature of love. Of all the qualities of God, the greatest of them, which encompasses everything, is love, which He showed to us by coming to the world in human form to die for our sins; to justify and sanctify us and make us more like Jesus. Love is the core of who God is, which means that the essence of who we are is love, and we need to be aware of this and embody it. 1 Corinthians 13:4-7 describes love and how to become a love being just like God.

> *Love is patient, love is kind. It does not envy, it does not boast, it is not proud. It does not dishonor others, it is not self-seeking, it is not easily angered, it keeps no record of wrongs. Love does not delight in evil but rejoices with the truth. It always protects, always trusts, always hopes, always perseveres.*

> *1 Corinthians 13:4-7 (NIV)*

When love flows out of you, you begin to flow out from a firm and grounded sense of identity.

Now repeat these affirmations and embody these statements that reveal who you are as a product of God created in His image.

Who Are You?

My Daily Beauty Affirmations

I am love, and I express love in everything that I do
and to everyone that I meet.

I am worthy of every good thing in the world. I am
worthy of a great life.

I am unique, and I bring my uniqueness into
everything that I do.

I am valuable; my work is invaluable. I add value
to humanity.

I am enough. I have everything it takes to be
significant and successful because I was a complete
product from God before He launched me into the
world.

I am beautiful inside and out because I see the best
in myself and others.

I am daring. I dare to dream and create a
masterpiece with God.

I am confident in God, who is my creator.
Therefore, I am a success.

I am bold, and I boldly serve the agenda of the
kingdom.

I am limitless, my potential is endless, and I can
accomplish anything that I choose.

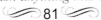

Who Are You?

I am deserving of a life full of wealth.

I am capable of doing all things through God who strengthens me.

I am magnificent because I am the daughter of a majestic God.

I am powerful, and I have the strength to control my life and circumstances.

I am courageous to manifest my visions. I am the woman for the job.

I am light. I cannot be hidden. Light radiates to the world through everything that I represent.

I am authentic. I serve my world with the authenticity of who I am.

I am strong and fit for all the different expressions of me in the different areas of my life.

I am brilliant, and I exude brilliance in everything that I do.

I am generous, and I give freely from the abundance of wealth that God has given me to promote His agenda.

I am talented. I recognize my talents and use them to serve the world.

I am fabulous. I do extraordinary things because I have an incredible father.

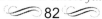

Who Are You?

I am gifted. I recognize my gifts, and I use them in the different spheres of influence God has placed me.

I am excellent. I have an incredible spirit; everything I do is outstanding,

I am awakened to what God is calling me to do in my generation.

I am joyful. I feel joy from deep within. The joy of the Lord is my strength.

I am a voice in my generation, preparing the way for the Lord.

I am free from everything masking my true beauty. I am open to becoming all that God has in store for me.

I am fearless. I completely embrace my fears because greater is He that is in me than he that is in the world.

I am audacious, daring, and unconventional as I operate in the kingdom anointing.

I am an inspiration, and I inspire people to become more because I have come in the volume of the books that God has written about me.

I am adorable. I am loved. I am a magnet for miracles.

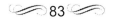

Who Are You?

I am optimistic about everything in my life. I know everything is working for my good.

I am empowered to carry out my vision to the extent to which God wants me to.

I am growing daily in spirit, soul, and body.

I am rich in love, wealth, and relationships.

I am expressive of everything God has placed in my heart.

I am amazing. I am a wonder to behold.

I am mindful of creating an atmosphere for God to reign on earth.

I am delightful. The joy of the Lord is my strength.

I am unapologetically me because I know who I am. I am a product of God.

I am thankful for all that I have.

I am ambitious about becoming all that has been written of me by God.

I am grateful for every blessing that God has and will create for me.

I am passionate about creating solutions to the problems God has called me to solve in the world.

Who Are You?

I am optimistic about the difference I am making in the world.

I radiate love, and others reflect love to me.

I am righteous to serve the vision God has placed upon my heart.

I am trustworthy, responsible, and compassionate.

I am flourishing in wealth.

I am creative energy in human form because I was formed in God's image.

I am refreshed daily by God's words.

I am intelligent. I reflect the intelligence of God.

I am wise. I reflect the wisdom of God.

I am kind to myself and other people.

I am whole and complete.

I am happy with my life.

I am wealthy because I have the gift of men, the gift from men, inner peace, gifts from God, and God's anointing.

I am blessed beyond measure with gifts and talents, and I use them every day.

Who Are You?

I am grateful because I was fearfully and wonderfully made.

I am self-assured in who I am in God.

I abide in my source, so out of my heart flows rivers of living water that will never run dry.

I am productive, just like my God. I do not hustle, but I do productive and meaningful work aligned with who I am.

I am complete in God.

My positive energy is contagious.

I influence to change my world positively.

I have abundance in every area of my life.

I listen to my inner truth as I connect with the spirit of truth - the Holy Spirit.

I have peace within me as I partner with God to create and impact the world.

I have fire in me to bring positive change to the different spheres of influence God has called me to.

I am a gift to the world.

I unmask my beauty daily to connect with who I truly am in God.

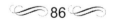

Exercise:

1. Write or print out the beauty statements that represent who you are.

2. Post them in a place where you can see them daily.

3. Repeat these statements daily and ensure you feel and embody these truths about yourself because this is who you are.

05: You Are Uniquely Wired

I t is amazing to know who you are and that you are unique and created in God's image; therefore, you have His branding embedded within you. So good!

When God created you in His image, He packaged you. You are a package sent to earth to deliver your gifts to your generation. Simply put, your gifts are part of who you are. You are your gifts! That sounds simple, but yes, you are your gifts.

Remember, I said that the question *"Who am I?"* always haunted me, and I struggled to get answers until I deliberately connected with God, who revealed the truth of who I was to me. He began to show me that who I am is also a combination of how He has uniquely wired me through everything He has deposited inside me. I like to call those deposits gifts. So, your gifts are those things that God has deposited inside you to guide you into fulfilling your purpose. Your gifts align you with the essence of who you are, who you have always been, and who you are becoming.

I love to picture myself as a large gift box beautifully wrapped with a custom-made tag with my name on it. If I just look at the gift box and do nothing with it, it will just sit pretty wherever it is and may even start to deteriorate. But if I decide to open it to see what is inside, I can read the gift manufacturer's manual and understand its use.

So, to understand your gifts, you need to read the manufacturer's manual. For instance, a motor vehicle comes with the manufacturer's manual on what to use it for, where to use it, and how to use it. Same as the gifts God has deposited in us, we need to partner with our manufacturer, God, to ultimately uncover and understand what to use our gifts for, how to use our gifts, and where to use them.

Understanding your gifts and their use is how you birth purpose, but first, let us identify the gifts that have your name on them. These gifts come as a combination of your personality, your strengths, your values, your passions, and your unique story. The realization of this combination helped me better understand myself and give myself to the world. I also created an acronym for the word 'gifts' from this combination.

G - *Genuine Passion*

I - *Innate Strength*

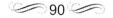

F - *Fundamental values*

T - *True Personality*

S - *Story*

In the following exercises, I will be walking you through the process of fleshing out your gifts by identifying the content of the gift that is you! Exciting times are here. Let us go!

G - Your Genuine Passion

Genuine passion is that inner nudge or energy that God has deposited inside you to pull you toward what you love and do naturally. It is that powerful or compelling emotion or feeling of desire for something; that rising excitement you feel is your genuine passion. Your genuine passion is not your purpose, but it is one of the unique gifts that serve as a cue to lead you into understanding your purpose.

Here are some questions to ask yourself to identify your passion.

Exercise:

1. What issues in the world do you feel strongly about? What problems in the world keep you awake at night?
2. What concerns, causes, or issues in the world occupy your mind consistently?
3. What is one topic you can talk about, research, or spend hours on without realizing it or getting bored?

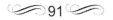

4. Is there a group of people you are drawn to or who come to you for advice?

5. Which organizations or ministries are you most drawn toward or involved with?

6. If you could spend an entire day doing something you love or enjoy? What would you do? Describe the day in detail.

7. What message do you have to share with the world?

8. If you could make a difference in one way, what would you do?

9. Who inspires you, and why do they inspire you? Who is it that you see and feel like they are living your dream life?

The first time I completed my passion exercise, I discovered that I had a strong desire to help women and girls develop their inner confidence to live fuller and more expressive lives. I especially hate to see women in abusive relationships or women not standing up for what they want in their relationships and career. Whenever I see a woman in an abusive relationship, it hurts me deeply, and I strongly feel like jumping in to help, but then I realize that the work must, first of all, be done from the inside. It is not an outside job at all. If women knew the power they carry, our world would be a better place. If we, as women, rise to who we are, we will make better choices in our relationships, raise better-behaved children, make more significant contributions at work, and generally make the world a better place.

I - Your Innate Strength

Your strengths are those innate natural abilities that God has deposited inside you to help you serve your purpose. Don Clifton, one of the authors of *"Now, Discover Your Strengths,"* has done extensive work to group human beings' strengths into thirty-four themes. In the exercise below, you will identify the top five strength themes that define you to develop and deploy them to serve your purpose.

#1 Achiever	*#13 Deliberative*	*#25 Learner*
#2 Activator	*#14 Developer*	*#26 Maximizer*
#3 Adaptability	*#15 Discipline*	*#27 Positivity*
#4 Analytical	*#16 Empathy*	*#28 Relator*
#5 Arranger	*#17 Focus*	*#29 Responsibility*
#6 Belief	*#18 Futuristic*	*#30 Restorative*
#7 Command	*#19 Harmony*	*#31 Self-Assurance*
#8 Communication	*#20 Ideation*	*#32 Significance*
#9 Competition	*#21 Includer*	*#33 Strategic*
#10 Connectedness	*#22 Individualization*	*#34 Woo*
#11 Consistency	*#23 Input*	
#12 Context	*#24 Intellection*	

From the above themes, I first highlighted ten strength themes that resonated with me, and I later narrowed them down to my top five strength themes: Activator, Adaptability, Developer, Positivity, and

Futuristic. These themes were the top five that described my natural abilities.

F - Your Fundamental Values

God has instilled His values in us from the beginning. Your values are the standards by which you want to live your life. The five most important values to you are your fundamental values. Just as organizations have values, individuals do too! You may have lots of values but narrowing them down to five helps you appreciate what is most important. Your values are unique to you; even if two people happen to have the same values, such as generosity, each person will demonstrate it differently in her daily actions and language.

Exercise:

- Using the above strength finder themes, highlight your top five strength themes.
- Write a list of the top ten things you enjoy doing, even if you do not do them right now.

Your top ten list says a lot about you. It reflects what feeds your spirit, and when examined closely, you can quickly determine your core values. Now let us go on a treasure hunt, searching for the jewels secretly embedded among your favorite activities. Go through your top ten list, and for every item, ask yourself, *"Why do I enjoy this?", "Why is this important to me?"* By asking these simple questions, your core values will shine through. You will have a chance to see them clearly and harvest them so that the entire world can see them too. Follow along as I do this for the items on my list. This will help you understand how to pull out the gems tucked neatly into the things that bring you joy.

See examples below:

1. I love to cook - It gives me a sense of creativity.
2. I love to spend time with my family - It gives me peace, joy, and happiness.
3. I love to host my friends - It gives me positive energy.
4. I love to learn by attending workshops & events - It gives me a sense of empowerment.
5. I love to read - It increases my knowledge capacity and grows my mind.
6. I love to talk/speak - It gives me a sense of expression.
7. I love to volunteer for activities that improve the lives of people - It gives me a sense of community and love.
8. I love to teach and transfer knowledge - It gives me positive energy, a sense of generosity, and deepens my spirituality.
9. I love to dance - It gives me a sense of freedom/independence, expression, and happiness.
10. I love recommending things I believe in and that have worked for me - It gives me a sense of love.

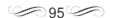

So, from my list of the top ten things that I love to do, I have answered the question - *"why do I enjoy this"* or *"why is this important to me."* This has helped me define my fundamental values as creativity, peace, joy, happiness, positive energy, achievement, knowledge, empowerment, perspective, expression, community, generosity, spirituality, growth, freedom, independence, and love. As much as everything on this list is important to me, I will narrow my fundamental values to five by grouping my values.

1. Joy (You can group happiness and positive energy under this.)
2. Peace
3. Freedom (you can group independence, expression, and creativity under this)
4. Growth (you can group knowledge and empowerment under this)
5. Love (you can group spirituality, generosity, and community under this)

It is that simple!

Note that although you are working from your top ten list, that does not mean you will end up with ten core values. You might end up with more, or you will find that some overlap or repeat. When you have completed the task, review your words, and cross out the duplicates. Your goal now is to condense your list into five ultimate core values. If there are many words and you are not sure how to whittle them down,

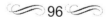

circle ten items that resonate with you. Then, see if you can narrow them down to five.

Here are some examples of core values:

Abundance	Honesty	Presence
Acceptance	Humor	Resourcefulness
Awareness	Imagination	Responsible
Beauty	Inspiration	Romance
Capable	Integrity	Security
Community	Inventiveness	Sensitivity
Compassion	Joy	Sensuality
Connection	Leadership	Serenity
Courage	Love	Sincerity
Creativity	Mastery	Spirituality
Energy	Minister	Spontaneity
Family	Open-mindedness	Strength
Freedom	Originality	Tranquility
Fun	Patience	Trust
Grace	Peace	Understanding
Growth	Persuasiveness	Uniqueness
Health	Playfulness	Wisdom

I now know that joy, peace, freedom, growth, and love are particularly important to me. The question I ask myself whenever I am about to make a decision in any area of my life is: *Does this align with my fundamental values? Do I feel joy, peace, growth, freedom, and love?*

As long as the answer is yes, I feel more confident in making those decisions.

Your fundamental values are a huge part of who you are. Once you identify them, every decision you make, every action you take should align with your fundamental values; if they do not, this is a red flag, and you may feel discontent with life. Your behavior, choices, and relationships all reflect your values. Honoring them is key to living a beautiful and authentic life.

T - Your True Personality

This term describes the traits a person consistently shows at different times and in different situations. Your true personality is how you show up and how you flow out into the world. It is your unique signature. Identifying your true personality makes you aware of it and ultimately guides you into nurturing it. This can also help you glean important insights about yourself and help you clarify your purpose.

Many psychologists have done extensive work on personality from online quizzes to online assessments, etc. I took the Myers-Briggs Type Inventory (MBTI) Personality profile. The MBTI was created by psychologists and has been used and studied by psychologists and businesses for decades. If you have ever been asked to take a personality test at your job, it was most likely the MBTI. Why would they want to know about your personality? For the same reasons as you—because your personality type can tell them a great deal about your natural talents, where you thrive, and who you will (and will not) get along with.

My results aligned perfectly with my strengths, and I could see myself in this beautifully thought out description.

My Personality

The driving quality in their lives is their attention to the outer world of possibilities; they are excited by continuous involvement in anything new, whether it be new ideas, new people, or new activities. They look for patterns and meaning in the world, and they often have a deep need to analyze, understand, and know the nature of things. People like me are typically energetic, enthusiastic people who lead spontaneous and adaptable lives.

Exercise:

- Go online and take your personality test and identify your true personality type and write out the description.

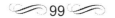

S - Your Story

Yes! Your story is part of your gifts, and until you start to see it that way, you are doing yourself and the entire humanity an injustice. Your story is unique to you, and it is not a secret to be kept. It is meant to be shared with others and liberate people. Your story is usually full of the messages God is sending you to share with the world. So, I want you to embrace the good, the bad, and the ugly parts of your story and begin to ask yourself what the message or the central theme of your story is. In your story lies your message to the world because no one on earth has had the same life experiences as you. So in this section, you will be pulling out memories from your childhood until now, and you will write your own unique story based on your experiences and lessons you have learned in life, be they good or bad.

Exercise:

Do a timeline of your life and gather stories:

- What memories stand out for you? Write down all the significant events you can remember and write about how you felt when the event happened. The memories may be good or bad; just write down as many as you can.

- Draw a table and group the seasons of your life as seen below; you can always customize these headings to your life stages. No two people have the same story. Own your story and be truly authentic to yourself. You can write as many stories as you can remember

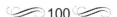

from each season of life. Also, write out the lessons that jump out to you from each story.

Elementary School	High school	University	Career	Marriage
Story 1	Story 1	Story 1	Story 1	Story 1
Story 2	Story 2	Story 2	Story 2	Story 2
Story 3	Story 3	Story 3	Story 3	Story 3

I have summarized a few of the memories that I felt were defining for me below. These are just some of my memory examples to get you into the storytelling mood. The idea is to write down everything you can remember.

Elementary/Primary School

I represented my school at a National concert for children, where I led the Nigerian National Anthem in French. I felt like a super-star!

High School

I started getting into trouble a lot around Grade 11 because I suddenly realized what I wanted to stand for. I hated rules, and I wanted independence and freedom. My high school was full of rules and regulations. I rebelled against the school authority, especially when I thought the rules did not make sense. I gradually found my voice and began to stand up for what I believed. I believed in girls' rights but did not know how to effectively deliver the message as I had no one to guide or mentor me.

University

In year 2 of Engineering School, I remember telling my friend that I was not interested in becoming an engineer. She asked me what I wanted to do, and I told her I would have loved to be a cosmetologist. She laughed and disregarded what I said because it did not make sense to her. She thought, how could someone in Engineering School want to become a cosmetologist? It did not make sense to me either, but that was what I wanted.

Career

I remember feeling on top of the world in 2014, when I became a project planning manager, managing a team of eight people, and reporting directly to the company's vice president. At that point in my life, I started to understand the power of the mind. I could become anything I wanted and achieve anything I proposed. I applied for that role based on a desire to become a manager in my field before my thirtieth birthday. I looked out for employment opportunities in that field, trained to get the necessary certifications that would qualify me for the role, and then I started applying. I got the job at the first interview I attended, and I was utterly blown away with the package they had for me. This was a goal that I set and manifested in just six months. My friends asked me how I was comfortable applying for the role, and I told them that as long as I could do 60-70% of a job, I believed that I was the woman for it. They all wondered at my confidence. I thought that was my dream job, but six to eight months into it, I began to lack motivation and frequently asked myself: *who am I?* I never received an answer, but I was determined to know.

Marriage

Earlier in our marriage, after the birth of our first child, we relocated to the UK, where childcare was costly. My husband was a trainee doctor, and I tried to secure my first job in the UK. My husband felt daycare was too expensive and that we could not afford it, and suggested that it may be wiser for me to look after our son and save money instead of getting a job, making money, and then using all that money to pay for childcare. I immediately told him that we would put our son in the best daycare we could afford and that I did not mind paying the fees with all that I would be earning. For me, it was not about money. It was about growing myself and being in a community of professionals. I wanted to be a present mom for my child while still building myself and my career too. The conversation went well, and I went on to start my first job in London. I did not want to be with our toddler all day with an absent mind thinking of all the things I could have been doing. I felt great that I was authentically communicating who I was to my husband.

Putting all your gifts together

After writing your own stories, identify the themes in them and the overall message that your story is telling.

Next, summarize all your gifts. Pull together each category in a similar table to the one below. This is what mine looks like.

Genuine Passion	Innate Strength	Fundamental Value	True Personality	Story (Message/theme from the story)
Women connecting to their identity.	Activator	Joy		Confidence
Genuine Passion	Innate Strength	Fundamental Value	True Personality	Story (Message/theme from the story)
Helping women address	Adaptability	Peace	Extrovert	Embracing who you are as a woman and

their mindset problems.				still having it all.
Empowering women to have it all.	Developer	Freedom	Intuitive	Love for the beauty industry, especially makeup.
	Futuristic	Empowerment	Thinker	A need to be authentic in every area of my life
	Positivity	Love	Perceiver	A strong conviction of my beliefs

After seeing all my gifts on the table above, I felt so powerful discovering the potential within me. I realized that if I could activate this potential and put it to good use, I would begin to embody even more of who God says I am.

06: Why Are You Here?

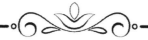

Now that you have greater clarity regarding who you are and have been able to identify your potential, the next question to answer is - *'Why are you here? – Why do you have all this potential?'*

Your potential is the vehicle that allows you to deliver your purpose. You need to activate your potential to step into your purpose, but first, let me introduce you to the world of purpose.

Author and speaker Myles Munroe said, *"When purpose is not known, abuse is inevitable."* You need to understand your 'why' or else you will abuse yourself, and people will also abuse you.

In the previous chapters, you identified the things that make you who you are. Hopefully, you now realize that it is who you are that powers what you do, where you do it, and how you do it. Given the different gifts you have identified, your purpose cannot be limited to just one thing as there are many different things that you can be. Therefore, your purpose is the central role you play in the world or the central theme running through everything that you do in every area of your life. For example, based on my identity as God's product and my gifts (my genuine passions, innate strength, fundamental values, true personality, and story); I find myself helping people, especially women, develop and activate their potential, so they can see what is possible when they lean into who they are. As I do this through different means, I would say that my purpose is not limited to just one thing.

In this chapter, I will be guiding you on how to write your purpose statement, which I also call your **"Personal Mission Statement."** A Personal Mission Statement reflects who you are, your passions, values, personality, strengths, and the message from your personal story. Before we dig deeper into writing our mission statements, there are some principles you need to know about purpose.

Principles of Your Purpose

Your purpose is co-creation - Purpose is your opportunity to partner with God to create something extraordinary. God's desire is for you to rule the earth for Him, for His will to be done on earth. This is called a kingdom agenda. Kingdom simply means the King of Glory dominating the earth. God's kingdom agenda is God's blueprint for how He wants us to live as His children here on earth and how He wants the world to operate. You cannot deliver purpose on your own. You need to partner with God, your manufacturer, to create something outstanding because your purpose is more significant than you.

Your purpose is inherent – What you need to serve your purpose has already been placed within you. In other words, your gifts are meant to help you fulfill your purpose.

Your Purpose is multi-faceted - You are wired with the potential to do many things, not just one thing. So, do not feel the need to confine yourself to doing one thing.

Your Purpose is interdependent - You are part of a bigger picture, so the world needs you and the purpose you were born for. Likewise, you also need others to fulfill your purpose. You cannot fulfill your purpose in isolation.

Purpose provides vision - When you have better clarity regarding your purpose, you start to see what is possible, and this is how you become creative.

I never saw myself as a creative person until I started living purposefully. I used to tell people that I was not a creative person; just show me how it is done, and I will do it for you but do not rely on me to create anything new. It is incredible how my story has changed. Now, I see creativity everywhere I go. I am now so creative with everything I do that I no longer need to see what other people are doing before I embark on a project, no matter how green the experience may be for me. I have a conviction of what I want, and I just go for it, whether it is uncharted territory or not. Same with my businesses, I do not follow the traditional model of researching my competitors. I have since left that competitive model, and I have started to create my own.

Dear Adoniaa Woman

This is the life I want for you—the peaceful life of creativity. Yes, creativity will stretch you but be rest assured that it will not stress you. What I genuinely want for you is a life where you are continually creating such that you do not have time for the competition. When you work with a clear purpose in mind, you show up every day feeling that you are part of something bigger.

I will use my gifts table from the previous chapter to craft a purpose and mission statement as an example to guide you toward crafting yours.

My Mission Statement

I partner with God to daily advance the agenda of the Kingdom by upholding my values of joy, peace, freedom, growth, and love in all that I do. I am filled with vitality and passion when I empower people, especially women, to activate and develop their potential. I feel content and enriched each day as I capitalize on my

positive energy and enthusiastic personality to lead people to live fuller and more expressive lives.

The first day I wrote this down, I felt so powerful. This was the beginning of my creative journey. This statement is power-packed and made me realize how to use all of who I am to create change and impact the world. Your purpose statement should highlight your values, passions, strengths, personality, and message from your personal and unique story. It should not restrict you but should enable you to create! It is a simple statement highlighting how you want to live your life going forward, and this is how you want to start to brand yourself. It is from your mission statement that different expressions of you will flow out.

Exercise:

Write your mission statement using this template:

I partner with God to daily advance the agenda of the Kingdom by upholding my values of (insert your fundamental values) in all that I do. I am filled with vitality and passion when (insert how you use your strengths to deliver your passions). I feel content and enriched each day as I capitalize on my (insert your personality and strengths) (insert your contribution and the impact of your contribution drawn from the message in your story.)

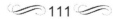

Stage 2 Summary:

I hope you will agree that this stage of self-discovery is an eye-opening one. How are you feeling now that you are beginning to gain better clarity about who you are? This is not a one-time process but a process you should go through from time to time to keep rediscovering yourself. The good thing is that you can start to partner with God to create an epic life with the truth you currently know about yourself. Are you ready? Let's go!

Stage 3 - CREATE

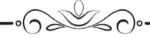

Conception

Becoming

Birthing

Everyone who steps into purpose becomes a visionary that carries a burden to create. Whenever you find yourself saying there is more to you, you can become a visionary who creates. Now that you have your purpose statement written down, it is time for you to partner with God to co-create a beautiful life, the life you were born to live.

When you know why you are on earth, you can begin to create visions around every area of your life, including the solutions you can bring to the world. This is not a one-time process. It is a process that you need to continually commit to because as you evolve, your vision will also evolve with you.

So, what is a vision? The Oxford Dictionary defines vision as the ability to think about or plan the future with imagination or a type of transcendent discernment. It is a mental image projecting what the future will or could be. It is something you can see in advance of the actual event.

Personally, the process of creating reminds me of the three stages of pregnancy:

The first trimester - I call it the vision Conception stage. In this stage of pregnancy, you have just conceived, and you are super excited. You are carrying the seed of your vision, but no one can see it. You must be so diligent in taking your pregnancy multivitamins. You are told to avoid certain medications that can potentially affect the seed you are carrying. Some tell friends and family; others wait for everyone to be pleasantly surprised. It is generally the stage where you have been implanted with seed, and you must carry that seed with diligence to prevent a miscarriage.

The second trimester- I call this stage Becoming. There is no more morning sickness. You are just beginning to show, but it does not mean it is time to give birth. People will start noticing that you're pregnant, even if you do not tell anyone.

The third trimester - I call this stage Manifestation. At this stage, it is obvious you are about to go through a birthing process. It is no longer a question of *"is she pregnant?"* Or *"is she not?"* You are heavy and ready to give birth.

07: Conception

"For as he thinks in his heart, so is he ..."
Proverbs 23:7a (AMP)

At this stage, you are super excited about the level of clarity you have about yourself and what you are to do on earth. Now you want to take it to the next level by visualizing your future based on what you know about yourself and what you can do with what you know about yourself. In this stage of conception, there are two things you want to do:

- *Visualization*
- *Creating your canvas*

Conception

A. Visualization

When you visualize doing something, your brain functions as if you are performing the task, so the brain does not distinguish between doing something and visualizing it. This is what makes visualization highly effective. You create a subconscious belief that the reality you have imagined already exists—and because of the energetic force of your beliefs, your life begins to align with that imagined reality. Trust me; this is what has happened in my own life. I have attracted everything that I focus on through visualization, and I want you to do the same.

The whole idea here is that your energy flows where your mind goes. In other words, your energy follows your attention, and your attention follows your focus. So deliberately focusing your thoughts on where you want your life to go targets your energy in that direction. Your visualization has energy, so as you visualize your intent, you will start to notice the energy surrounding it, leading to miracles and eventually bringing your vision into existence.

Visualize the thing that you want. See it. Feel it. Believe in it. Design your mental blueprint and begin to create. Live and act as if what you desire has already occurred by replaying the mental image. This will then attract the desired experience into your life.

Exercise:

Where do you see yourself in the five different areas of your life (*Health, Self-image, Relationships, Career, and Finances*) identified in your life

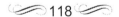

assessment in Stage 1? As you consider each area, keep in mind your mission statement so you can flow out of your core into the future you desire for your life. Write your history now!

Health

Mind

- Write down your mental and emotional health strategy.
- Write down how you want to feel daily

Body

- If you were always getting adequate rest, how will that routine look? What time would you go to bed? What time would you get out of bed? How would it feel?
- What would an ideal fitness program look like for you? What would you do, and when?
- What would an ideal eating pattern or nutrition lifestyle look like for you?
- What is your ideal weight?
- What are your physical health and medical checkup strategies?

Spirit

- How do you want to incorporate 'me' time into your daily, weekly, monthly, and yearly routine?

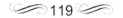

- Do you engage in regular character and personal development activities?
- Describe a spiritually enriching moment you want to build into your daily, weekly, monthly, and yearly routine, such as prayer, meditation, or worship.

Self-image

Self-esteem

- How do you want to enrich your mind to feel a good sense of self-worth daily?
- How do you feel about your appearance and wardrobe selections?
- What steps are you taking to accurately represent who you are?

Attitude

- What steps do you want to begin to take to develop a positive outlook on life?
- How would you love your friends and family to describe your attitude?

Appearance

- When you look in the mirror, do you feel beautiful?
- Do you feel you have an authentic style?
- How do you want to be perceived when others meet you?

Conception

Relationships

Romance

- What would an ideal relationship look and feel like?
- What is your love language? What is your communication style or preference?
- What is the ideal dynamic of your relationship? (What do you expect from your spouse?)
- What kind of person do you want to grow old with?
- Describe your ideal date night.
- Describe the things needed to keep your marriage healthy.
- What mutual hobbies and interests do you have?
- What goals do you have together (especially after your children leave home)?

Children

- What type of relationship do you want to have with your children?
- What values do you want to pass on to them?
- Where do you see your children in the next 5, 10, 20 years?

Extended Family

- What type of relationship will you love to have with your extended family (parents, in-laws, sisters, brothers, aunties, and uncles) if you do not already have it?

Friendship

- What kind of close relationships do you need to develop?
- Do you have a mastermind group (a peer group for brainstorming, mentoring, and support)? If so, who are those people?
- What does your support system look like?
- Whom do you value more than anyone else?
- Who values you the most?
- Who holds you accountable for your decisions?
- What relationships have encouraged your gifts to flourish?
- Who challenges you with next-level thinking?
- In whom can you confide?

Career/Calling

- If you knew you would not fail, describe the work you would do.
- What sphere of influence have you been called to?
  - Home or Family

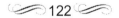

- o Religion/Church/Ministry
- o Business & Economy
- o Government & Politics
- o Arts & Entertainment
- o Academia & Education
- o Media
- o Law & Justice
- o Science &Technology
- o Sports
- o Fashion
- o Social Reformation

- What is your ultimate dream job?
- What industries do you want to work in?
- What would you like to achieve?
- What would you do even if you did not get paid for it?
- What does your ideal career look like?
- Do you want to work from home?
- Do you enjoy being around people every day?
- Do you love being on the road?
- Describe your career path in detail?
- What are the steps you need to take to get there?
- Out of these twelve spheres of influence, which sphere is God calling you to work in?

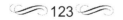

Finances

Imagine all your financial needs and goals were met. What would that look and feel like?

- How were you able to achieve that?
- What would a workable budget look like? Do you need to make some revisions to your current one (or create one)?
- Describe your retirement plan. How much do you want to retire with?
- Describe your saving and investment plan.
- How do you plan to underwrite your vision?
- Describe your investments and assets, including intellectual property, real estate, and other portfolios.

B. Create Your Canvas

After going through visualization, you also want to begin to see that mental image by creating your canvas. There is so much power in what you fix your eyes upon- such as a vision board that enables you to focus your view on a particular outcome you want to create because whatever you focus on grows and what you think about expands. This is a powerful principle because whatever occupies your mind will ultimately determine the types of decisions you make every day. This is why a vision board is such a powerful tool for aiming your focus in the direction of your dreams.

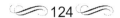

Conception

A vision board is your canvas of future possibilities. In this visual representation, images of what you want to see manifested in your life are gathered together in one place so that they can be reflected consistently. It could be a bulletin board with push pins, a poster board where you paste images with a glue stick, an online Pinterest board, or whatever works for you, as long as you can see it daily. The vehicle used to visually display your dreams and desires is not as important as where you place it.

Your vision board must be positioned somewhere you will see it repeatedly, be it on your bedroom wall, office wall, bathroom mirror, or in your closet, or hallway—wherever it will catch your eyes daily.

The key is to prominently display a collection of images of what you want your life to look like in the future. It is all about what you continually see with your eyes and your mind. Being able to see what your conscious mind desires to achieve will help your subconscious mind go to work on your behalf to make it possible, again *'As a man thinketh in his heart, so is he'* - Proverbs 23:7.

Assembling your vision board is merely creating a blueprint or template for your envisioned future. It is the framework you will use to begin manifesting your dreams into reality. Find pictures representing or symbolizing the experiences, feelings, and possessions you want to attract into your life, and place them on your board. Have fun with the process! Use photographs, magazine cutouts, pictures from the Internet—whatever inspires you. Be creative. Include not only pictures but anything that speaks to you. Consider including photos of yourself on your board. You may also want to post your affirmations, inspirational words, quotes, and thoughts here. Choose words and images that inspire you and make you feel good. Use only the words and images that best represent your purpose, your ideal future, and inspire positive emotions in you. There is beauty in simplicity and clarity. Too many images and too much information will be distracting and harder to focus on.

Here's My Simple 6-Step Process for Making Empowering Vision Boards with Soul.

Step 1: Start with your mission statement.

Write down your mission statement on a paper and pin it to the center of your vision board. This will ensure you create a vision that aligns with your values and all that you are. It will also ensure that your vision is part of something bigger and that it benefits others.

Step 2: Begin with the end in mind.

You already visualized what you want, so bring out the journal where you wrote down everything you visualized and start transferring it to your vision board. Start gathering pictures of how you want each of those five areas of your life to look. Search for visual representations of the transformations you would like to see in each area. Just by being awake and aware, you will begin to see images of what you are hoping for.

Step 3: Collect a bundle of old magazines with beautiful pictures or print from the Internet.

If you are not a magazine reader or currently do not have any magazines at home, ask your friends to give you any magazines they no longer want. You should also be able to pick some up for just a dollar or two per magazine at your local thrift store. Or just search on the Internet.

Step 4: Find pictures that represent your goals and inspire you.

Schedule a couple of hours one evening or weekend to go through the magazines and cut out pictures representing your vision or use pictures from the Internet and use Canva or Pinterest to create your board.

Fun tip:

The last time I did my vision board was for the *Adoniaa online Teen Beauty Camp*. We called it a vision board party and turned up the radio, so we had a little musical party going on as we cut out our images, which made it very vibrant and fun.

When looking for images in magazines or on the Internet, look for those that immediately make you say, *"Yes! That is what I want in my life!"* They do not have to be physical objects or literal interpretations of what you want in your life. Instead, focus on how the images make you feel. I remember my first vision board—I had a picture of Oprah speaking to many women. I put that picture on my vision board because I wanted to start speaking at women's events. This is now a reality, so I have updated my board's photos with personal photos of me speaking at events for women.

Step 5: Add affirmation words that represent how you want to feel

I like to add words to my vision board that describe how I want to feel daily such as: *"I am joyful," "I am abundant," "I am powerful," "I am fearless," "I am loved," "I am strong," or "I am healthy."* You can insert your beauty affirmations on your vision board in an attractive way.

Step 6: Take a few moments to pray over your vision board every day

To get the full benefit from your vision board, you must place it somewhere you can see it every day; so that you can pray over your vision board at least once or twice a day, so your goals are top of mind as you train your mind to attract what you truly want into your life. As you pray over your vision board daily, the Holy Spirit will begin to download how to manifest it to you. You can also review it every night before you go to bed to prompt your subconscious mind to develop new ideas for achieving your goals while you are sleeping. That way, you wake up in the morning bursting with motivation to succeed, and you are far more likely to notice and act on opportunities that will bring you closer to your goals.

Your Vision Statement

Your vision statement should stem from your mission statement to reflect a more significant purpose beyond you.

A vision statement should be:

- *Simple and clear*
- *Actionable*
- *Focused on the effect you will have on others*
- *Expressed in affirmative language that resonates with you*

Format of a Vision statement

To…………. So that…………..

The first blank represents the contribution you make to the lives of others. The second blank represents the impact of your contribution.

I have shared my vision statements for the different areas of my life below to give you some examples of what to include on your board.

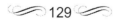

Self-image - Based on your mission statement, what will your self-image look like to enable you to fulfill your purpose?

To deeply love myself and see myself as a highly valued product of God that has been created in His image and likeness so that I can fully become the woman to deliver God's kingdom agenda.

Health - Based on your mission statement, what will your health look like to enable you to fulfil your purpose?

To be sound in my spirit, soul, and body so that I can be fit for the work God has called me to do.

Finances - Based on your mission statement, what will your finances look like to enable you to fulfill your purpose?

To live in abundance and wealth by intentionally accessing and experiencing wealth in all its entirety so that I can advance God's kingdom agenda.

Relationships - Based on your mission statement, what will your relationships look like to enable you to fulfil your purpose?

To understand the role of each relationship in my life and maximize the potential of all my relationships so that the world can be a better place.

Conception

Career - Based on your mission statement, what will your career look like to enable you to fulfill your purpose?

To develop, validate, equip, and inspire people, especially women, to connect to their true and unique identity at every stage of their lives so they can live fuller and more expressive lives.

EXAMPLE OF MY VISION BOARD PHOTO

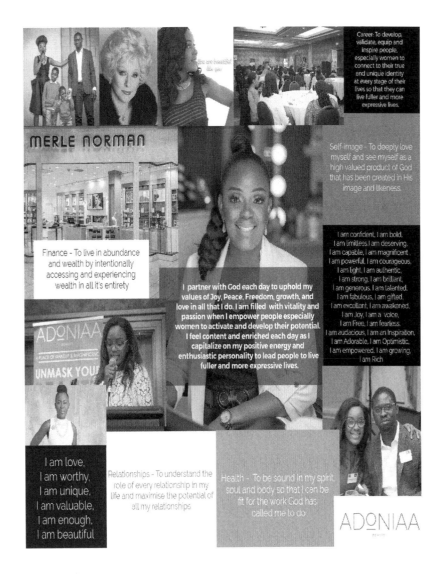

My Vision Board Summary

The photo on the previous page is a summarized version of my vision board as of 2020.

I have put Mary Kay's photo on my vision board because I love the woman she was, her beliefs, and the company she built based on what she believed. I have included Merle Norman's beauty studio because I love their business model, and that is where I am taking *Adoniaa Beauty*. I have placed my family's photo on there because they are my world, and they matter so much to me, so nothing I do must compete with the quality time I spend with them. I have also placed my mission statement, vision statements, and affirmations all over the board. I've included photos of me speaking to women. And I've put a power photo of me in the middle representing the more polished version of me as I daily commit to polishing all my gifts into becoming the woman God has created me to be.

The vision board exercise is one you want to review yearly and update the board as you begin to dream bigger and get more precise on your assignments.

Conception

Exercise

Write out your Vision Statement

- Create your vision board using my 6-step process above.

- Look at your vision board and the images you collected representing how you want your life to look in the five areas discussed above.

- Describe in your own words how life would currently be if it is what you envisioned for each of the five areas.

- Write a vision statement for the five different areas of your life (*Health, Self-image, Relationships, Finances, and Career*), then display your vision statements on your vision board and speak those words upon your life daily.

- Put the affirmations from chapter 4 on your board or any other affirmations that speak to you and declare these words over your life daily.

08: Becoming

This part of the Create stage can be likened to the second trimester of pregnancy, which I call 'Becoming.' At this stage, you are already showing, but you have not birthed yet. People are beginning to see you evolve and say things like *"You have changed, you are evolving, I love what you are doing ..."* because you are already looking like the carrier of your vision.

The first time it occurred to me that I was becoming the person on my vision board, which I love to call personal branding, was in 2017. I was beginning to embody the woman I had visualized, and it was noticeable to my friends and family. I had called my friend to wish her a happy birthday when she told me how proud she was of me building a personal brand. Before then, I had never heard the term personal branding, so I went to check out the meaning on Google. I found out that personal branding meant being consistent in showing the world your personal beliefs and what you stand for through your different expressions, be it a career, business, ministry, etc.

More people began to say the same thing, and I also started getting invitations to speak on personal branding. By the time I got some clarity on who I was and discovered the central theme in my life that gives purpose to all of who I am, I began to represent my brand in everything I did, and people started noticing. People that knew me before started saying they were loving how I was evolving, and people that were meeting me for the first time instantly connected emotionally with what I stood for.

You see, darling, you are first the vision! The journey to manifesting your vision starts with you. It is *being* before *doing*, meaning *"it's your evolution first before manifestation."* It is who you are becoming first before you start to manifest anything. You do not need to tell people who you are before they know. You just simply radiate it by flowing out of your core! Discovering who you are and aligning with it will naturally set you up to become that person representing her brand in every area of life. If you want to attract success and prosperity, you must make your brand authentic to who you are.

This is your opportunity to be aware of your uniqueness enough to infuse it into everything you do and finally share your uniqueness with the world. Never be afraid of the qualities that set you apart and draw attention to you because people who stand out from the crowd, defy the odds, and accomplish great things. There is no one with the exact composition of your core makeup. Even if you have an identical twin sister, there will be personality differences, experiential differences, and so many other differences. This uniqueness is your superpower in every area of your life. Be unapologetic about it, and see it as your opportunity to embody and give voice to your vision.

I used to think the word 'branding' was only associated with business, and I know most people associate branding with business. When building a traditional business, you are mostly told to create a brand identity for your business based on what your ideal clients want, and you are often asked questions like - *"Who are the people in your target market?" "What are they thinking?" "Where are they shopping?" "What is their lifestyle like?" "What is the perception that you need to create to appeal to your target audience?"* You will then be advised to build a brand identity around your target audience's tastes and personality. Right?

Well, personal branding is the exact opposite of that. In personal branding, you want to flow out from your core into everything you do. This is the first business you want to build an identity around before building any other business.

I call it, "Me, incorporated." You want to build a strong personal brand for yourself by mastering yourself so powerfully that other things you create will start to flow from who you are.

I started to build my brand based on my Mission and Vision statements. I only work on projects I have a genuine passion for so that everything I do comes from my heart. I also started to leverage my strength at work and in my relationships. I ensure that my values are aligned with everything I do. I stopped apologizing for being extroverted and exuding positive energy because I know that is part of who I am. I also leverage my story by sharing it through speaking and writing to encourage people to live fuller and more expressive lives.

Branding yourself into the woman you are becoming is the most authentic way to live life, whether you are an entrepreneur or a career woman. A great example of a woman who is clear about who she is and her vision is former First Lady of the United States of America, Michelle Obama. Michelle Obama's branding was so attractive, and that made people connect emotionally with her. She instantly became America's sweetheart because she became her vision. When she left the White House, after eight years as First Lady, Oprah interviewed her and asked her how she could carry herself with so much grace ... Michelle said she just decided to be true to herself and worked only on projects close to her heart. Michelle Obama is a visionary who has branded herself personally beyond being the First Lady of the USA. That is why even after leaving the White House, she keeps inspiring us all.

Another excellent example of a woman who branded herself with her vision is the late Mary Kay Ash, founder of Mary Kay Inc. She founded Mary Kay Inc. based on her personal beliefs and vision that women can have it all. She brought her dream to life through Mary Kay Cosmetics by empowering women through coaching and training to build a vision and become the woman who manifests the vision. The world is waiting for your uniqueness. Make it attractive and serve it hot like you genuinely know who you are.

Exercise:

Imagine someone is reading your autobiography (*your bio*) in the next five years. What will it sound like? Who will you have become based on the compelling vision that you carry?

Now, write your biography based on how you see your future self, using your Mission and Vision statements as guides.

After writing it, start to embody it in every area of your life.

Example of my Bio

Adedoyin Omotara is a kingdom wife to an amazing man she fondly calls Babyluv, and the healthy mom of two boys (she calls them her nations). She is a beauty entrepreneur, women's empowerment advocate, speaker, life coach, and business coach. Her passion for living a fuller and more expressive life made her leave her successful corporate engineering career to become a beauty entrepreneur and women's empowerment advocate.

"Unmask Your Beauty" - *Embrace your soul essence- Let your inner light shine! This is the powerful mantra behind everything that*

Adedoyin does. Adedoyin has built a successful multinational beauty company through her franchise program and keeps on inspiring women to do more and be more. She sits on the board of many female-owned companies and has built a platform for women to equip them to embrace the higher calling of God upon their lives.

I wrote the first two paragraphs in 2017 when I had never been invited to speak anywhere or mentored or coached anyone. But fast-forward to three years later—I have been invited to speak at numerous women's events, and I have mentored and coached women in business and life. I have entirely embodied the woman in the first two paragraphs of my bio. I recently updated my bio by adding a 3rd paragraph, which includes the woman I see myself evolving into in the next 1-3 years. This journey is an evolutionary journey, and nothing is set in stone. You will get to update your bio as you evolve. This is the joy of every transformation and life upgrade that you experience, realizing the truth that there is more, and you can become more of who God wants you to be if you completely surrender yourself to the process.

09: Birthing

At this stage, you are heavy and fully ready to give birth and bring forth. You are about to leave the ordinary behind for a life of greatness. I call this stage Birthing. Birthing is essentially bringing something tangible into your life. It takes an attitude of grit, perseverance, and mental strength, just like how you feel when you are close to delivery. The contractions, the pains, the water breaking, the pushing are all part of the process.

You are only as strong as your courage, convictions, and determination to make this move and take this step despite the bumps, cramps, turns, and collisions along the way. It does not matter whether you fly, run, walk, creep, or crawl. If you take steps toward birthing your vision, you will eventually collide with your best days, waiting just beyond the zone of discomfort and disappointment.

You do not birth what you want. You birth what you have conceived and believed.

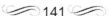

Below, I will share three elements that have helped me birth the different expressions of my vision:

1. Goal setting with soul
2. Designing an effective life system
3. Mobilizing people

1.Goal Setting with Soul

Goals are your visions broken down into smaller, manageable action plans. To achieve any goal, you need to have a clear vision of what you want to achieve and where you are heading. This is what will determine everything else you do with your time. A clear vision is required to achieve your goals. In creating goals with soul, you will use your vision statement and vision board to create your goals. Your goals must align with your vision. Manifesting your goals is you manifesting parts of your vision. Once you master that art, you will see your vision coming together nicely.

When setting goals, you need to ensure that you empower your goals, or else, your goals will not happen. To empower your goals means to set smart goals. That means that they must be:

1. Specific
2. Measurable
3. Achievable
4. Realistic
5. Time-bound

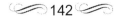

A particularly good example of setting a smart goal with soul is the writing of this book. When I set this goal in April of 2020, I wrote an action plan that looked like this:

> *I want to write a book titled "Unmask Your Beauty" to empower women on their self-discovery journey. The book will be launched on October 31, 2020, meaning that the manuscript must be ready by August 31. I am aware that I have a full life as a visionary, a deliberate mom of two young & active boys, a homemaker, a present wife, friend, sister, and full-time entrepreneur. However, I will achieve this goal by waking up at 5 am every day to spend my creative hours, which are the first three hours of my day on it. Once the manuscript is complete on August 31, the book's publishing will be outsourced so I can focus my time on creating a launch team that will help promote the book until the launch date of October 31.*

Let us break down this acronym using my example.

Specific - Your goal should be soulful and specific. It must be sensible, simple, and significant to your vision. The goal of writing a book called *"Unmask Your Beauty"* is very clear and significant to my overall vision. What you want to achieve must be clear; some goals are just confusing or unclear, and that is why they fail. To ensure your goal is specific, ask yourself the following questions:

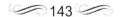

- *What do I want to accomplish?*
- *Why is this goal important?*
- *Who is involved?*
- *Where is it located?*
- *Which resources or limits are involved?*

Measurable - Your goal should be measurable. When you look back, can you say you gave this goal 100%? You need to be able to track your progress when you evaluate your goals. The launching of my book is how the achievement of my above goal will be measured. The day I launch my book is when I can check off my goal as completed, and I can then move on to other pursuits.

Achievable - Your goal should stretch your abilities but remain possible to achieve. A goal is achievable if the 'how' of accomplishing it is identified, and it also considers the season of life you are in.

In my goal action plan, I recognized that I had a full life but specified how I would achieve it by waking up at 5 am and dedicating three hours of my day to it, even with my full life.

Relevant - A goal must be relevant. This step is about ensuring that your goal aligns with your vision. Is it making you that woman who can carry the vision? Is it linked to your vision? The goal I shared above is linked to my vision of empowering women to live fuller and more expressive lives. For me, it is another avenue to reach out to more women. Ask yourself the following questions to ensure that your goals are relevant to your vision.

- *Does this seem worthwhile?*
- *Is this the right time?*
- *Does this match my other efforts/needs?*
- *Am I the right person to reach this goal?*
- *Is it applicable in the current socio-economic environment?*

Time-Bound - Every goal needs a target date, a deadline to focus on, and something to work toward. My goal had two dates on it; the first was the time to complete the manuscript, and the second was the date to launch the book, so I was very clear on the dates, which will ensure that I can track when the goal is completed.

2. Designing an Effective Life System

The example above where I broke down the action plan for my book has been a goal since 2017, but I kept disempowering the goal by not making it smart until April 2020 when I finally decided to empower it. This can happen to many of the goals that you set if you do not empower them. There are so many other goals I have disempowered like that, and that really made me realize that you do not get results by merely setting goals, but you only get results by your everyday habits based on the system you have in place for your life. Trust me; you have a system you are currently operating on. The question is - *Is that system serving you? Is that system able to carry your vision? Is the system strong enough to carry you into the future you want?*

Simply put, if you do not like your results, go back and look at your systems. I do this every time I cannot manifest my vision for the different areas of my life. Author James Clear wrote in his book, Atomic Habits - *"You do not rise to the level of your goals, you fall to the level of your systems."* In other words, focusing on designing an overall system that aligns with who you are becoming yields better results than merely setting goals. Having an effective life system is really what helps you manifest your goals and, in turn, helps you manifest your vision.

So how do you design a system for your life? Through your everyday habits—those little habits you cultivate in your daily life to become a woman who achieves her goals. Your life today is essentially the sum total of your everyday habits.

A system is a process for predicting the achievement of a goal based on specific, orderly, and repeatable principles and practices. It leverages your time, money, and abilities and is an excellent tool for personal growth. Systems are deliberate, intentional, and practical. They work—regardless of your profession, level of talent, or experience. They improve your performance. A life without any systems is a life where the person must deal with every task and challenge from scratch.

If you want to make the most of your personal growth by getting the most you can out of every effort and doing it as efficiently as possible, you need to develop systems that work for you. That will be a personal thing because your systems need to be tailored to you. For a system to be effective, you must put the following into consideration.

A. Take Your Vision into Account

One of my favorite quotes is from Stephen Covey in his book, 7 Habits of Highly Effective People, where he stated - *"We may be very busy, we may be very efficient, but we will also be truly effective only when we begin with the end in mind."*

When I started creating systems for my personal growth, I was very, very intentional. Besides having a commercial beauty studio, I knew that I would be speaking, leading my staff, coaching, mentoring, writing books, taking my kids to their activities, etc. My efforts had to support and advance my abilities in those areas, so I ensured that I trained my staff on all services, and I also ensured that all processes were documented so that I do not have to be at the store all the time.

People who excel, regardless of their profession, develop systems to help them achieve the big picture. It is not enough to be busy. If you are busy planning, busy reading books, and busy going to conferences, but they are not targeted on the areas essential to your success, you are not helping yourself.

What is your big picture? In what areas must you grow to achieve your purpose? What systems can you develop to advance yourself in those areas, and every day?

B. Maximize Time

A system is of little help to you if it does not consider your priorities.

Brian Tracy, in his book *Time Management* says, "Perhaps the very best question you can memorize and repeat over and over is, *"What is the most valuable use of my time right now?"* Your answer to that question should shape any system you create for yourself. You should also ask yourself, *"When is my most valuable time?"* because you will always want to make the most of it. For me, it is mornings after dropping my kids at school. The first 2-3 hours are my most creative time. When I recognized that, I started to time-block my weekday mornings to do creative work and ensure that I do not book clients or any meetings at those times. What systems do you need to put into place to help you maintain your priorities?

C. Measure the Results of Your System

An effective system will give you your desired results. If you are not getting the results you want in your life, you probably have a faulty system, and you want to fix that. Do not be reluctant to adjust systems you develop or even abandon them if they do not serve you well. However, you may want to try out any system you develop for at least three weeks (the usual time needed to start developing a positive habit) before evaluating its validity.

D. Be Consistent

Ensure that your system is one that you can easily repeat regularly? The consistency of this pattern of habit is really what makes it a system.

3. Mobilize People

People are crucial to the manifestation of your vision; they are an indispensable resource for fulfilling your vision. You need to be able to identify the type of people that can help you accomplish your vision. I call them Visionary Partners. Our vision is usually bigger than us, and there are people God has placed in our lives or that God will put in our lives to help us fulfill that vision. Our work is to identify our Visionary Partners carefully. There are different roles that different Visionary Partners play on our visionary journey. I will highlight some that I have seen play out in my life. It is also useful to know that some people can play more than one of these roles in your life.

A. **The Collaborators:** When I started the *"Unmask Your Beauty"* conference, I saw it as an opportunity to collaborate with other visionaries that believed in my message and saw it as a training ground for *Adoniaa women* to start their visionary journey.

   The conference gives every woman speaking an opportunity to share her story, inspire someone, and have a sense of ownership toward the event. This conference is sold out every year in Calgary because these amazing women believe in the vision and carry such a strong conviction for the vision, thereby influencing people in their network or community to attend the event.

B. **The Financiers:** These are people that will believe in your vision so much that they provide financial support to make it happen. I have often had sponsors for the *"Unmask Your Beauty"* Conference, Teen Beauty Camp, and many other expressions of my vision. People believe in it and decide to sponsor the programs. It is completely mind-blowing, but it is so real.

When people hear a compelling vision and believe in it, they always want to be a part of it.

C. **Strategists:** These are people who, when you share your vision with them, they immediately get it and can bring your vision to life with their expertise. For example, I met my digital marketing guy called Sylvester in 2016, and all I did was tell him about my compelling vision. Since sharing my vision with him, we have partnered to create masterpiece ad campaigns, marketing, and sales campaigns that reflect my brand's true identity. Often, I just give him a brief, and he produces a masterpiece from it. He just gets the vision and always delivers value.

Coaches and consultants fall into this category because they use their wisdom, skills, and expertise to bring your vision to life.

D. **Industry Leaders:** Industry Leaders give you a foot in the door. I remember connecting with Evelyne Nyairo, founder of *Ellie Bianca Beauty,* when I started *Adoniaa Beauty*. She had started her business before me, and I adopted her as my mentor. She opened doors for me that I would never have been able to open

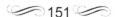

by myself. She gave me access to other go-getter businesswomen in Calgary that have helped elevate my business in Calgary.

E. **Volunteers -** People who believe in you and love your vision will want to serve you without pay. They are not interested in the money because they are entirely sold out to the vision. I have volunteers that reach out to me yearly for the Teen Beauty Camp that *Adoniaa* organizes and the *Unmask Your Beauty* conference.

F. **Co-workers** - Co-workers bring their technical and administrative skills to help you deliver your vision. You must invest in them by training them and continually telling them about the big picture so they can represent your brand effectively.

G. **Your Audience - The Crusaders:** These are people who follow your work, buy your products and services, believe in your compelling vision so much that they also become crusaders for your work. Your best crusaders are people that you serve by understanding their pain points and offering them solutions. They believe strongly in your vision and will tell the whole world about you.

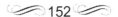

All these people are critical to the manifestation of your vision, and you must identify and nurture these relationships with respect.

Stage 3 Summary:

At the Create stage, you have started to see and birth what is possible in your life. The good news is, there is always more—as long as you stay connected to your source and embrace a growth mindset, you will have better clarity about yourself, and your vision will keep getting sharper.

Stage 4 - **GROW**

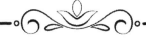

Grow Yourself
Grow Your Mind
Grow Your Influence

Y ou need to be intentional about growing yourself, as no one will do this work for you. I became intentional about my personal growth by continually improving myself. In this section, I will be taking you through some elements of self-growth that have personally worked for me.

Personal growth is how a person recognizes herself as valuable and, therefore, continually invests in developing herself to reach her full potential. At this point, I trust that you believe that there is so much value within you to give to the world. You are an amazing woman, and the world is waiting for your manifestation.

The process of continuously birthing your vision will require you to grow and stretch creatively, but such growth will only happen if you allow it and are intentional about it. Otherwise, you will often find yourself getting stuck and feeling too discouraged to carry on.

On my growth journey, I have discovered different versions of me, and I look forward to discovering even more as I evolve into the woman God wants me to be.

The creative work of vision can be very stretching, and in the process of undergoing this stretching, I have discovered three areas that you need to grow intentionally.

- Grow yourself
- Grow your mind
- Grow your influence

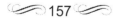

10: Grow Yourself

With the vision I had, I knew that I needed to invest in the right environment to cultivate this vision, so I invested in mentoring by joining the Super Working Mum Academy community. More recently, I joined the Immerse Inner Circle Community. In these two communities, we read personal development books together, pray together, and have monthly masterclasses on different life areas such as family, career, spirituality, relationships, parenting, etc., and ultimately grow together as a community. Being in a community where everyone is growth driven helped me not feel alone on this journey, as the visionary journey can sometimes be lonely if your friends and family do not get your vision. These groups have also held me accountable for all my goals and helped me achieve many short-term goals through various mastermind sessions.

Invest in Mentors

I believe we all have our different teachers in the different seasons of life that we are in; they may be younger or older than us or even in the same age group as us, but the key here is to identify your teachers per season to help you on your growth journey.

How Do You Know Your Teachers/Mentors per Season?

You can know who your teachers are by identifying the people who inspire you either online or in person. Anytime you see these people, you feel they are living your life, you see your future self in them, and you see how your values align with theirs. They may not have the same strengths or personality that you have, but you see yourself in them from their way of life and the type of results they are getting in their lives. Their definition of success is like yours, and you find yourself just loving everything about them.

As an intentional visionary, you want to find a way to connect with this individual or these people by doing some or all the following:

- Read books they have written
- Take courses they have created
- Subscribe to their podcasts
- Join their coaching communities
- Sign up to be on their email list
- Join their mastermind program if they have one

And basically, just find a way to connect with them as much as possible through their published work.

I have had different mentors at different seasons of my life. One of them is Tara Fela-Durotoye, popularly known as TFD. TFD has been someone I have always admired since connecting with her business in 2008, but I only started following her closely when I started *Adoniaa* and joined Instagram in 2015. Anytime I come across her work and all the things that she represents; I see myself in her. From her spirituality being the operating system of her life to her people-loving personality, to the way she empowers women, the joy she exudes, her value of having meaningful relationships and building them, her love for kingdom marriages and parenting, the principles she built her business on and so much more. I just really see aligned values and often see my future self in her. She does not know me, but she has always been a virtual teacher and mentor to me. So, what did I do to connect with her? I joined her email-based inner circle, where she shares nuggets of wisdom in different areas of life. I bought her course on how to structure a business, which has helped my own business. I follow her podcast, I attend her live webinars, and follow her closely. She has not written a book yet, but if she writes a book today on any topic, I will buy it. My point here is that being intentional about your growth lies in your hands. You need to know precisely what you want and go all out for it. I still look forward to the day I will meet TFD to tell her about her impact on my life, but I was intentional enough to learn from her through the different resources she has made available.

Detola Amure is another woman who inspires me through her way of life. Detola is the leader of Super Working Mum and a very sound productivity coach. I met her at a time of my life when I was confused about how to move forward with my vision, and I was also overwhelmed with balancing family life and work life. I signed up for Detola's coaching program, and she was the first person to open my eyes to the world of personal development and living a life by design. She helped me design a life system that worked in line with my vision without trading what truly mattered to me. I am still a member of her inner circle called Super Working Mum Academy, and this group has been instrumental to my continuous development.

As I began to grow, I started desiring to birth more expressions of the woman in my purpose statement, and I knew that I needed to step into a new dimension of me. Debola Deji-Kurunmi, popularly known as DDK, was the woman I felt could mentor me to step into this newer level. I love how she expresses different versions of her assignment while still tied to her purpose. She is the Queen of Multi-Influential flow, meaning you are not created to do just one thing, according to her, that is a gross underutilization of your potential. I agree with this ideology as I have different expressions of me, all stemming from my purpose statement that I want to manifest. She believes that we all have different expressions we can create from having a deep understanding of what our purpose is. DDK is a woman that manifests everything she represents with so much ease, and I wanted to learn how to manifest all my different expressions with ease too, so I enrolled in her coaching program, and my growth has never been the same since then.

I am sharing these stories so you also can start being intentional about your growth by identifying your mentors and learning from them.

Invest in Personal Retreats

Another proven way to grow yourself is to intentionally recharge yourself by investing some time in personal retreats. A personal retreat is a fantastic way to recharge and set your life in a new direction. Personal retreats give you space to rejuvenate, recharge, recollect yourself, and allow you to reflect, gain new insights, and access innovative solutions. They feel good on your mind, your body, and your soul. The process of manifesting your vision can stretch you as it has to do with giving yourself, your time, and resources, so you need to be intentional about refilling yourself and recharging your batteries.

How Do You Retreat?

You want to start your retreat by connecting with your source without any distractions and meditate, journal, read, etc.

Connect & Communicate with God

During your retreat, your main goal is to block out all noise and connect with your God, who is your source of strength, wisdom, knowledge, understanding, and everything that you are. This is your ideas factory where you receive fresh insights about your vision. You can connect and communicate with God all day by ensuring that your spirit is in tune with Him but clearing out sometime in your calendar to focus on Him alone is a powerful tool for personal growth. Your spirituality is the operating system of your life that can radically help you in your evolutionary journey, so you want to pay attention to this. You can connect to God through:

- Worship – Worship shows a lot of love and adoration to God by singing praises to Him and calling Him all the beautiful names. Just really loving upon God.

- Prayer - Prayer is communicating with God and pouring out everything in your heart to Him.

- Fasting - This is when you deny your body its physical needs to move the focus away from your body and toward your faith and spirituality. You can deny yourself food, sex, social media, etc. and just focus on connecting with God.

Meditating

According to Wikipedia, meditation is a practice where an individual uses a technique—such as mindfulness or focusing the mind on a particular object, thought, or activity—to train attention and awareness, and achieve a mentally clear and emotionally calm and stable state. I do not just want you to focus on any random object, but I want you to focus on the truth, which is the word of God. The scripture is God's prophecy upon your life, and until you start to meditate on it by focusing your mind on it, you may not manifest that prophecy.

"Finally, brothers and sisters, whatever is true, whatever is noble, whatever is right, whatever is pure, whatever is lovely, whatever is admirable—if anything is excellent or praiseworthy—think about such things."
Philippians 4:8 (NIV)

Meditation gives you better clarity about who you are and how you are supposed to serve your vision to the world. It also helps you recondition your mind daily to think the thoughts of God upon your life.

Journaling

Journaling is simply putting down your thoughts, experiences, and feelings on paper or in a notepad. It is an immensely powerful process that can help you date yourself again and become best friends with yourself. Since I started keeping journals, I have become more aware of who I am, and I am generally better able to respond to situations. If you are new to journaling and are not sure what to write, you can write about your day, including your thoughts, feelings, problems, challenges, upsets, joys, successes, and dreams, e.g., what do you notice, what are you thinking about, how are you feeling or what's the best part of your day/week.

How to Get Practical with Your Retreats

You can do your retreats daily, weekly, monthly, quarterly, and yearly. Of all these retreat routines, the daily retreats are the best way to incorporate a growth culture.

- ***Daily retreats:*** I incorporate daily retreats into my everyday routine because if you are waiting for a weeklong holiday in a quarter or a year before taking a retreat, you will break down and not perform optimally. A daily culture of growth requires you to be energized daily to work on your vision. You can work your retreat into the first hour of your day when you wake up or the last hour of your day before you go to bed. I prefer mornings, as that is when I am the sharpest. You can decide to choose whatever works for you. You can incorporate retreats into your daily routine by dedicating about thirty minutes to one hour in the mornings to meditating on the word of God, journaling, and spending quiet time with the Holy Spirit to simply listen.

- *Weekly Retreats:* You also want to dedicate a day in a week for yourself to spend more time in prayer and worship. This is the day you also want to invest in yourself by reading books and simply just be so that you can regain your strength.

- *Quarterly/Yearly Retreats:* This is the type of retreat you can do quarterly or yearly where you temporarily leave behind the usual distractions we all face for a time long enough to allow relaxation and for an inner change to occur. Setting aside time alone to be quiet and disconnect from the "normal" world is something we all need in this fast-paced world. We might not have realized it but stepping away from our phones for just a few minutes can be exceedingly difficult. Our spirit needs quiet, so you need to be deliberate about recharging yourself.

11: Grow Your Mind

As a visionary, you must embrace a growth mindset to see even bigger pictures of your vision and evolve into the woman who manifests the vision.

Carol Dweck did a brilliant job of defining a growth mindset and a fixed mindset. She says: *"A growth mindset creates a passion for learning rather than a hunger for approval. Why waste time proving over and over how great you are when you could be getting better? Why hide deficiencies instead of overcoming them? Why look for friends or partners who will just shore up your self-esteem instead of ones who will also challenge you to grow? And why seek out the tried and true instead of experiences that will stretch you? The passion for stretching yourself and sticking to it, even (or especially) when it is not going well, is the hallmark of the growth mindset. This mindset allows people to thrive during some of the most challenging times in their lives."*

I have highlighted four ways to grow your mind based on my own story:

Embrace your fears

When I got the vision to lead women on a journey of unmasking using a beauty platform, I was so confused as to how to merge the two because some people are even of the school of thought that makeup masks real beauty, so I wondered how a makeup company would lead women to unmask their beauty. I thought of it for several months, and I was almost going to give up on pursuing that vision because I had not seen anyone do anything like that in the beauty sector before. I thought to myself – *Doyin, just focus on providing services, selling products, and building a makeup school.* That's what I saw a lot of makeup and beauty brands doing anyway, so why did I want to complicate things? I knew my vision was different from this, but I had seen so many other entrepreneurs manifest it. This vision led me into uncharted territory, but I decided to embrace the fears and create a completely new path and story for my brand. The first breakthrough came when I started praying to God for clarity. He told me to change the names of my products to descriptions of who God created women to be, and I immediately obeyed. This clarity made the vision more compelling, and I became more confident to walk this path. Embracing a growth mindset of working my vision, not minding if I failed in the process, has turned me into a creative that has birthed more than ten expressions and counting just from one compelling vision. *Adoniaa Beauty's* vision is to be a globally respected beauty brand that uses the platform of beauty to uplift, validate, equip and empower women at different stages of life to connect to their true, individual, and unique beauty, and live fuller, more expressive lives. From this vision, we have created over ten expressions pointing back to this one vision:

- **Beauty Services** (Makeup detailing, Eyelash extensions, Waxing, Threading, Microshading, Microblading, Lash lift & tint, Facials, Hair, Nails, etc.)

- **Beauty Products:** Skincare – cleansers, toners, moisturizers, serums, masks, exfoliants, and Cosmetics – foundation, powder, eyebrow pencils, eyeshadow, eyeliners, mascaras, lashes, lipsticks, blushes, etc.

- **Beauty Academy** (Certifying people to become makeup artists and Aestheticians)

- **Partnership with *Adoniaa Beauty*:** We carry a local, black-owned beauty product in the store to build a strong local community, which is a vital part of our values.

- *"Unmask Your Beauty"* **interview series**

- *"Unmask Your Beauty"* **conference**

- *"Unmask Your Beauty"* **short films**

- **Teen beauty Camp**

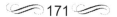

- **Women's Beauty Camp**
- ***"Unmask Your Beauty"*** book
- ***"Unmask Your Beauty"*** **Coaching Community**
- ***"Unmask Your Beauty"*** **Mastermind**

This experience simply taught me that a compelling vision has more than one way it can be expressed because it is usually bigger than you. You need to surrender to the process of growth and embrace your fears. Growing your mind is switching on the creative portals in your mind to accommodate what is coming. You need to expand and grow your mind to accommodate your vision's bigger picture as it comes to you. More can be done if you carry a compelling vision that connects with who you are. All that is required of you is for you to surrender and evolve with the process.

1. Challenge your mind, stretch out of your comfort zone

The mind is like a muscle that needs to be worked out, just like the body. Growing your mind is a very gritty process and requires a lot of learning and unlearning. When we started to plan the ***"Unmask Your Beauty"*** Global Conference 2020, my coach kept asking me how many people I wanted to attend the conference, and I just felt well I am sure to get 100-150 people to show up at the conference. Before the 2020 conference, I always had a yearly ***"Unmask Your Beauty"*** conference in Calgary, Canada, where we hosted about 100-150 guests, so that number was in my comfort zone as I had mastered how to work it. My coach kept reminding me to think global and decide how many people I wanted because that number was critical to the successful planning of the conference. It was so challenging to get my mind to grow into having thousands of people at my online conference basically because I already knew how to work a guest list of 150, and it had become comfortable for me. I decided to face my fears and plan for 1000 people. This changed how we promoted the conference, but I am thankful for the growth mindset that I embraced in making this happen. To grow your mind, you will have to stretch and come out of your comfort zone.

2. Accept failure as feedback

When I opened the first *Adoniaa Beauty* studio, I had issues recruiting the right staff. I had employed people whose values did not align with my company values, so the first year was spent turning over staff rapidly. I also recruited more staff than I needed, and so it was difficult to break-even. We were making money, but the overhead was so high. It just really seemed like I had failed in the business already in less than one year. I had seen other businesses like mine closing down because of this same problem, but deep down, I knew the problem could be fixed, and it was only a steeper learning curve for me. I took a one week break to reflect, and I came back with a plan because I knew that quitting was not an option. I opened the store to build a vibrant community of *Adoniaa* women who could get all their beauty services provided in one place. I learned from my mistakes and decided to restructure the recruitment process to not overeat into the overhead. What happened to my business in the first year of opening was enough to close the business, but I had to see that experience as a learning opportunity. As part of our current growth plan, we have a documented recruiting process that does not affect the business revenue.

3. See challenges as opportunities and relish opportunities for self-improvement

At the start of COVID-19, when I had to close the *Adoniaa Beauty* studio, I took the first week to reflect on what I wanted to do as we did not know when we would open again. Thankfully, the government made provision for my staff to get paid until we could open again. I saw that period as a time of retreat, while many people expected me to be anxious. I got calls from all over the world asking how I felt about closing *Adoniaa Beauty*, and my response to everyone was the same. It was sad to close the store because of the many women we physically connect with daily. But I reminded them that *Adoniaa* was not the store and that we will still connect with *Adoniaa women* through our online operations. That mindset helped me get highly creative, and *Adoniaa Beauty* did even better in terms of reach, influence, and revenue during the COVID-19 pandemic. Some of the things we did to pivot were:

In the past, we had hosted the *Adoniaa* Teen Beauty camp at the *Adoniaa* studio in Calgary, which could only accommodate six girls at a time. With the reality of COVID, we had two options:

- Option one: to cancel the camp for the year 2020.
- Option two: to embrace a growth mindset and set up an online camp.

Of course, we went with the online route, which required a lot more work regarding marketing and set up, but we could reach more girls and help them on their transformational journey into confidence.

I had always wanted to write the ***"Unmask Your Beauty"*** book because it is part of the vision, and it is pivotal to the growth of *Adoniaa women*. But I never really empowered the goal because I was so busy with the studio activities. It was not the vision I had for myself, but it took forever to detach myself from store activities and focus on the bigger vision. COVID eventually got me into that flow, and as soon as the lockdown started, I wrote it down as one of my goals and empowered it by making it a smart goal and working with a coach as my accountability partner. As a result of this, even after the lockdown, I am not tied to being at the store 24/7. I have specific days of the week on which I do not go out, so I can focus on other aspects of the vision.

I also had time to work on some courses I had always wanted to create for immigrant women in beauty. Many immigrant women ask me to guide them with starting their beauty businesses, especially in product creation. I had done lots of research in this industry even before I started

Adoniaa Beauty. Of course, it is the industry I am currently playing in, so I saw the lockdown period as the best time to create the course and make it accessible to them. The thank-you messages are still coming in from the women who attended the free webinar and the main course. This was tied to my vision statement to help equip women to step into their power.

I am sharing all these stories to encourage you that nothing in this world can take away your compelling vision as long as you embrace a growth mindset. Your compelling vision is greater than you, and it is not tied to any location. You are the vision, and if you are evolving, your vision will evolve into several expressions regardless of the situation in the world.

12: Grow Your Influence

Sociologists tell us that even the most introverted individual will influence 10,000 people during his or her lifetime. Everyone influences someone. That means the question we should all be asking is: How do I increase my influence?

Influence is earned. It does not come instantaneously, and it does not come by accident. So, we must be intentional with how we approach growing our influence.

There are two types of people: those who give value and those who receive value. Influence is always gained by providing value. When you become a

Everyone is a leader because everyone influences someone.

Adedoyin Omotara

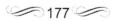

value creator, you begin to influence your world.

Now, there are only two questions to be answered: *"Will you choose to grow your influence?"* and *"Will you use your influence to serve the world?"*

As I continued my growth journey, I discovered that people wanted to connect with me; to learn and listen to my message. Are you teaching, training, sharing, equipping, and inspiring? Are you in a legacy-building season focused on helping others go to a deeper, greater level in their lives? Are you launching new ideas and creating initiatives, solutions, businesses, and charitable movements, all while using these avenues to share broader life lessons learned along the way? How do you increase your chances of helping others and making a significant contribution in your lifetime?

Author John Maxwell says, *"Think of yourself as a river instead of a reservoir."* Most people who do make personal growth part of their lives do it to add value to themselves. They are like reservoirs that continually take in water but only to fill themselves up. In contrast, rivers flow. Whatever water they receive, they also give away. That is the way we should be as we learn and grow. That requires an abundance mindset—a belief that we will keep receiving. But if you are dedicated to personal growth, you will never experience scarcity and always have much to give. John Maxwell lives out the principle of giving value by doing five simple things every day:

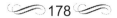

- *"Every day I Value People – If I don't value people, I'll never add value to people.*
- *Every day I think of ways to add Value to People.*
- *Every day I look for ways to add Value to People.*
- *Every day I do things that add Value to People.*
- *Every day I take inventory for 10 minutes.*
  - *Who did I add Value to today?*
  - *Who did I serve today?*
- *Every day I encourage others to add Value to People."*

I have adopted this plan and have seen tremendous growth in my influence. But this process does not happen overnight, it is an intentional act to create value and give value continuously, and it grows in stages.

Visually, it looks something like this:

- Level 1: Model
- Level 2: Motivate
- Level 3: Mentor
- Level 4: Multiply

Let us look at each level as we learn how to grow our influence.

Level 1: Model

Stanford University published a study titled "How We Learn." Their findings revealed that 89% of people are visual learners, 10% are auditory learners, and 1% learn by using their other senses.

Based on these findings, we know that leadership is caught, not taught! Suppose you want to have a significant impact on other people's lives, in that case, you must work alongside them so they can see your influence in action. The moment I decided I would grow my influence, I knew that I had to become my message first to lead by example and model my beliefs with my own life. Since then, I have inspired hundreds of other people that have connected with me to live in the identity of who they are. I see how my beliefs have influenced those around me over the past three years. I see it in my staff members, husband, children, extended family, friends, clients, and everyone I interact with, through my business, or any other avenue.

Meet Adoniaa Woman, Mosope

Mosope is a health and fitness coach with a compelling vision to educate, equip, and empower moms. Her vision is for women to stay healthy during pregnancy and postpartum and continue to get back to doing the things they love.

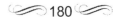

Mosope believes that, as moms, we can only thrive at taking care of others when we put our health and fitness needs first. Mosope is growing her influence in the health and fitness industry by modeling that it is possible to have kids and still care for ourselves. She believes that we need to be strong and healthy to play our roles efficiently, happily, and pain/issue free as moms. She daily models this belief system by sharing videos on social media of her exercise routine with her children often in tow. It is not unusual for her kids to join in on the (exercise) fun; after all, it is play. In doing this, she shows us how to involve our kids in our daily exercise routines- setting an example and instilling in them the importance of movement and exercise.

She inspires me. I tell myself that if Mosope, a mom of three kids under eight, can incorporate movement and exercise into her daily lifestyle, I have no excuse.

Level 2: Motivate

You become a motivational influencer when you encourage people and communicate with them on an emotional level. This process creates a bridge between you and others while also building up their confidence and sense of self-worth. When people feel good about themselves when they are with you, your level of influence increases significantly. The moment I started becoming the woman in my vision statement, opportunities to motivate people with my message began to open up. I have since spoken on many platforms and co-authored a few books to encourage people to step into their power.

Meet Adoniaa Woman, Eugenia

Eugenia is the founder of *Eleora Beauty*, a beauty company founded basically out of her pain, which she eventually turned into purpose. Eugenia's daughter, Eleora, went through a stem cell transplant, and as part of her treatment, she had to undergo chemotherapy. Eleora lost all her hair because of the chemotherapy. Eugenia tried to boost her daughter's confidence by mixing ingredients to create natural hair products to help her daughter's hair grow. These products helped to grow Eleora's hair, and she decided to share the products with the world as a way of inspiring hope in women at all stages of life. Eugenia is influencing women by motivating them to rise above their challenges and preaching hope to women at all life stages through her brand *Eleora Beauty*.

Level 3: Mentor

Mentoring is pouring your life into other people and helping them reach their potential. The power of mentoring is strong. As you give yourself, you help others overcome obstacles in their lives. You show them how to grow personally and professionally, and you help them achieve a whole new level of living. You can genuinely make a

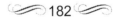

difference in their lives. I have mentored several women to start heart-centered businesses stemming from their brand because I believe that is the only kind of business that gives true fulfillment, which is truly built to last. It is always a privilege to influence people with the wisdom that God has given us. It comes from a mindset of abundance, knowing that the source of wisdom will never run dry. It also comes from a place of genuinely wanting to empower other people to step into their power. Trust me, people are looking for access to the wisdom you have cracked. Package your wisdom today and begin to offer it to people who need it.

Meet Adoniaa Woman, Eno

Eno had a compelling vision before relocating from Nigeria to Calgary. Her dream was to change the narrative of immigrants living abroad to live the lives they truly desire. Before Eno landed, she started researching the career of Business Analysis in Canada. She began writing exams to certify her to work in the field. Eno did not have it all rosy when she arrived in Canada. Her bags got lost during her connecting flight, and she lost all her belongings. Shortly after she landed, she got a job in her desired field. She applied to become a lecturer at one of Canada's most prestigious universities. Eno started making her dream a reality and, in no time, became popular among the immigrant community as the newest immigrant from Nigeria, pulling her weight in Canada. Eno noticed that many immigrant professionals who should have well-paying jobs struggled to make ends meet and worked odd jobs just to survive. She decided to carry other immigrants along by mentoring them on how to land their first professional jobs as well. Within two years of arriving in Canada, Eno has grown her influence by mentoring over 5000 immigrants through her mentoring and coaching programs. No wonder she has received several awards and accolades globally for being a change maker and mentor. Eno has been recognized by Forbes, RBC Top 75 Immigrants, Canada's 100 Most Powerful Women, and Women of Inspiration Awards, to name a few.

Level 4: Multiply

The highest level of influence you can have in others' lives is at the multiplication level. Many leaders struggle to make it to the fourth stage of influence, but everyone has the potential.

As a multiplying influencer, you help people you are influencing become positive influencers in others' lives. They pass on what they have received from you, as well as what they have learned on their own.

Mary Kay Ash is one of my favorite forerunners in the beauty industry. I had learned a lot about the principle of multiplication from her business and her life story, which she documented before she died. Mary Kay Ash's compelling vision was birthed out of the pain she felt from the memories of the opportunities denied her in her career because she was a woman. She decided to build a company where women will not be held back, a company where women would be allowed to pursue unlimited opportunities. She transferred this belief system into every beauty consultant, and it is just so contagious. If you meet any Mary Kay consultant, you will know that they are selling empowerment and using makeup as a platform. Everyone who interacts with her business and everything associated with her instantly catches that dream of greatness in everyone and that you can have or be anything you want. The Mary Kay dream is still alive in every Mary Kay consultant today as if she were still alive herself. That is the beauty of intentionally multiplying yourself.

I have consistently modeled my beliefs about the power that women carry and have intentionally motivated and mentored hundreds of women in the past three years to step into their power and live a fulfilled life.

My next mission is to multiply this dream with the Franchising model, where *Adoniaa women* can own their *Adoniaa Beauty* franchises and start to build their community of *Adoniaa women* in different cities of the world.

This is my dream, to see every woman step into her power and become all that God has created her to become. *Adoniaa* is the revolution of beauty.

Stage 4 Summary

Growth never ends, and this is the stage where you have to remain for life as personal growth is what will set you up on a constant journey of mindset reconditioning, personal rediscovery, and higher levels of creation. You should embrace a flowing sense of self, whereby you are perpetually reframing, reorganizing, rethinking, rebirthing, and unmasking yourself.

Exercise:

In what ways can you start to create value for people in your tribe?

Epilogue: About Adoniaa

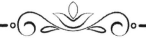

To write a great book, you must first become the book. That is why this book is *Adoniaa's* story intertwined with my own life story of transformation and, of course, the revolutionary stories of many *Adoniaa women* that I have had the privilege of connecting with.

Our story is not about money, status, or fame. It is the story of every woman that is ready to step into her power. *Adoniaa* is much more than a company; it is my dream in action. A movement to empower every woman to step into her power!

The beauty industry embodies a diverse, nimble, intimate, and empowered space. As a beauty brand, *Adoniaa* will support women to shape their beauty from within. The *Adoniaa woman* is self-assured and exudes confidence, kindness, intelligence, joy, and gratitude. Her individual beauty, expressed from the inside out, is elevated with *Adoniaa* cosmetics and skincare products.

Adoniaa is not selling a specific image or ideal, but rather a viewpoint on what true beauty looks like: *an empowered woman.*

Makeup as a Platform for Empowerment

At *Adoniaa*, skincare and makeup are the microphones for the brand's empowering message. Skincare and makeup play vital roles in women's preparations to meet each day confidently. Women can create their lives as much as they can make up their faces. Makeup truly empowers individuality. It is the ultimate vehicle for self-expression. At *Adoniaa*, confidence becomes visual.

Why Lipstick Is at the Forefront of Our Brand

- Thoughts lead to words – a woman's lips are the last place her thoughts reside, and they are vital to direct the actions and decisions that follow.
- A woman has several opportunities throughout the day to apply lipstick—in these moments, she can remind herself that she can choose her thoughts and how she defines herself.

Epilogue

Adoniaa's Vision

Adoniaa's vision is to be a globally respected beauty brand. To use the platform of beauty to uplift, validate, equip, and empower women at different stages of life to connect to their authentic, individual, and unique beauty and live fuller and more expressive lives.

Adoniaa's Values

- We believe in supporting individual dreams
- We stand behind quality and create best-in-class products and services
- We believe in joy and laughter and taking a loving approach
- We are accessible to all
- We strive for simplicity
- We believe in the power of community

The *Adoniaa woman* finds true beauty when:

- She shares her gifts with the world
- She does what she was created to do
- She expresses love
- She sees beauty around her
- She believes in the magic of a new day
- She pursues things that fill her
- She chooses to be grateful

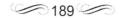

- She makes herself a priority
- She sees the best in people
- She makes peace with her fears
- She shows up as her authentic self
- She gives up judging herself and those around her
- She loves herself
- She unmasks her worth, strength, and power

The Face Behind *Adoniaa*

My name is Adedoyin Omotara. I created *Adoniaa* to empower women to define their own beauty. My vision for *Adoniaa* will be realized when women worldwide celebrate who they are, no matter their shape, size, age, or skin color. When women stop comparing themselves to each other and any type of ideal assigned to them by the media or their culture, my work will be complete.

I chose skincare and makeup because the practice of applying these products is a meditative ritual. In the morning, during skincare and makeup application, I want women to hear my message: *they are beautiful, unique, powerful, and strong.* With the simple act of applying blush or mascara, I want to remind women that only they get to define who they will be that day.

Every time women apply lipstick throughout the day, I invite them to remember their morning intention to be self-possessed.

Epilogue

In the evening, skincare is a practice that prepares for reflection and rejuvenation. I want to be the voice that reminds women that no one can assign beauty at all hours of the day—women define that for themselves by embodying who they are. Real, lasting beauty has roots in love, peace, joy, generosity, courage, kindness, and gratitude. Inner beauty radiates. It is the only beauty constant. Inner beauty grows. Inner beauty is timeless. Inner beauty is confidence and power. True beauty does not come from the outside. It comes from the inside out. *Adoniaa* is my touchstone—it is a name rooted in the Phoenician language that has a combined meaning of '*goddess,*' '*ruler,*' and '*beautiful woman.*' This is my vision—for all women to realize that this is within them.

Yours in beauty & truth

Adedoyin Omotara

Your Next Steps

s we conclude, I would like to encourage you not just to read this book, get excited, and then go back to your old ways of thinking and living an average life. You are a visionary person, and I will love for you to take the next innovative steps.

It is likely that you still have questions or need more guidance to identify what action steps you should be taking. You may need clarity on discovering who you are. You may need support to manifest your vision, or you may just want to plug yourself into a community that can help with your personal growth.

If that is you, I would love to walk alongside you on your journey by inviting you to join the *"Unmask Your Beauty"* Online Community.

Your Next Steps

The *"Unmask Your Beauty"* Community has been designed for women to receive continuous support. The online community provides access to numerous personal development masterclasses, coaching, e-books, and masterminds. The objective is to help women continuously evolve and manifest their compelling vision. Go to www.unmaskyourbeauty.ca for more details. Come join other *Adoniaa women* and me as we unmask our beauty and become all that God has in store for us.

Endnotes

Introduction

- Marianne Williamson, A Return to Love: Reflections on the Principles of "A Course in Miracles"
  Publisher: HarperCollins (March 15, 1996)

Stage 1: Awaken

Chapter 2: Identifying Masks

- Impostor syndrome (n.d.). In Wikipedia. Retrieved October 25, 2020, from https://en.wikipedia.org/wiki/Impostor_syndrome
- Napoleon Hill, Think and Grow Rich
  Publisher: TarcherPerigee (August 18, 2005)

Stage 2: Discover Yourself

Chapter 4: Who Are You?

- Image defined. Dictionary.com. Retrieved October 27, 2020, from https://www.dictionary.com/browse/image?s=t

Chapter 5: You Are Uniquely Wired

- Don Clifton, Now Discover Your Strengths
  Publisher: Gallup Press (January 29, 2001)
- The Myers & Briggs Foundation. Myers Briggs Type Indicator instrument. https://www.myersbriggs.org/my-mbti-personality-type/mbti-basics/

Chapter 6: Why Are You Here?
- Myles Munroe, Understanding the Purpose and Power of Woman
  Publisher: Whitaker House (July 1, 2001)

Stage 3: Create
- Vision defined in the Oxford Dictionary. Retrieved October 27, 2020, from (https://www.lexico.com/definition/vision)

Chapter 9: Birthing
- James Clear, Atomic Habits
  Publisher: Avery (October 16, 2018)
- Stephen Covey, 7 Habits of Highly Effective People
  Publisher: Free Press (November 9, 2004)
- Brian Tracy, Time Management
  Publisher: AMACOM (January 20, 2014)

Stage 4: Grow

Chapter 10: Grow Yourself
- Meditation (n.d.). In Wikipedia. Retrieved October 26, 2020, from
  https://en.wikipedia.org/wiki/Meditation#:~:text=Meditation%20is%20a%20practice%20where,emotionally%20calm%20and%20stable%20state.

Chapter 11: Grow Your Mind
- Carol Dweck, Mindset
  Publisher: Ballantine Books (December 26, 2007)

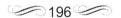

Chapter 12: Grow Your Influence
- John Maxwell, The 15 Invaluable Laws of Growth
  Publisher: Center Street (October 2, 2012)
- Stanford University Study
  (https://ed.stanford.edu/news/stanford-scholars-untangle-science-learning)

UNMASK *Your Beauty*

join the movement

share your story

www.unmaskyourbeauty.ca

Manufactured by Amazon.ca
Bolton, ON

29422800R00118